Julien Delarocque

Metabolic profiling of hyperinsulinemic horses

Cuvillier Verlag Göttingen
Internationaler wissenschaftlicher Fachverlag

Bibliografische Information der Deutschen Nationalbibliothek
Die Deutsche Nationalbibliothek verzeichnet diese Publikation in der Deutschen Nationalbibliografie; detaillierte bibliographische Daten sind im Internet über http://dnb.d-nb.de abrufbar.
1. Aufl. - Göttingen: Cuvillier, 2021
Zugl.: Hannover (TiHo), Univ., Diss., 2020

Nonnenstieg 8, 37075 Göttingen
Telefon: 0551-54724-0
Telefax: 0551-54724-21
www.cuvillier.de

1. Auflage, 2021
Gedruckt auf umweltfreundlichem, säurefreiem Papier aus nachhaltiger Forstwirtschaft.

ISBN 978-3-7369-7426-5
eISBN 978-3-7369-6426-6

University of Veterinary Medicine Hannover

Clinic for Horses

Metabolic profiling of hyperinsulinemic horses

THESIS

Submitted in partial fulfilment of the requirements for the degree

DOCTOR OF PHILOSOPHY

(PhD)

awarded by the University of Veterinary Medicine Hannover

by

Julien Delarocque

Nogent-sur-Marne

Hannover, Germany 2020

Supervisor:	**Prof. Dr. Karsten Feige**
Supervision Group:	**Prof. Dr. Karsten Feige** **Prof. Dr. Klaus Jung** **Prof. Dr. Korinna Huber**
1st Evaluation:	**Prof. Dr. Karsten Feige** Clinic for Horses, University of Veterinary Medicine Hannover, Foundation, Hannover, Germany **Prof. Dr. Klaus Jung** Institute for Animal Breeding and Genetics, University of Veterinary Medicine Hannover, Foundation, Hannover, Germany **Prof. Dr. Korinna Huber** Institute of Animal Science, Faculty of Agricultural Sciences, University of Hohenheim, Stuttgart, Germany
2nd Evaluation:	**Prof. Dr. Heidrun Gehlen** Equine Clinic, Department of Veterinary Medicine, Free University, Berlin, Germany
Date of the final public defense:	26th October 2020

Parts of this thesis have been published or presented previously:

Publications in peer-reviewed journals:

Delarocque J, Frers F, Huber K, Feige K, Warnken T. **Weight loss is linearly associated with a reduction of the insulin response to an oral glucose test in Icelandic horses.** BMC Veterinary Research 2020;16.

Presentations at conferences:

Delarocque J, Frers F, Huber K, Feige K, Warnken T. **Effectiveness of weight loss in reducing the insulin response to a carbohydrate challenge.** 16th World Equine Veterinary Association Congress, Verona, Italy, 04/10/2019.

Delarocque J, Frers F, Jung K, Huber K, Feige K, Warnken T. **Plasma metabolome of horses during oral glucose tests.** 12th Congress of the European College of Equine Veterinary Medicine, Valencia, Spain, 20/11/2019.

Delarocque J, Frers F, Jung K, Huber K, Feige K, Warnken T. **Plasma metabolome of horses during oral glucose tests.** 4th Global Equine Endocrinology Symposium, Gut Ising, Germany, 08/01/2020.

Delarocque J, Frers F, Huber K, Feige K, Warnken T. **Weight loss in combination with physical activity is highly effective against insulin dysregulation.** 4th Global Equine Endocrinology Symposium, Gut Ising, Germany, 09/01/2020.

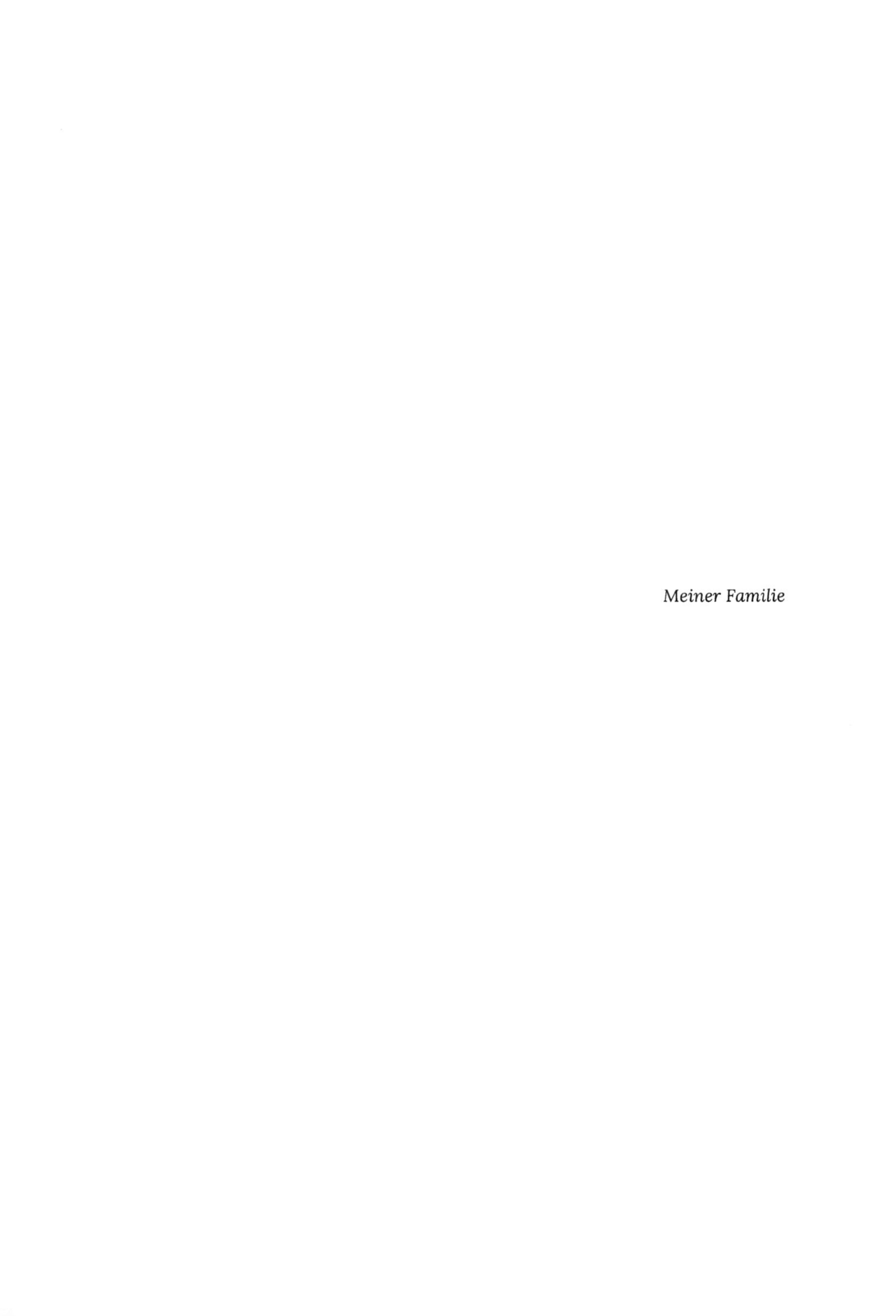

Meiner Familie

Table of contents

List of abbreviations

ACTH	Adrenocorticotropic hormone
Arg	Arginine
AUC_{ins}	Area under the curve of insulin over time
BC	Before Christ
BCS	Body condition score
C0	Carnitine
C2	Acetylcarnitine
CGIT	Combined glucose insulin tolerance test
CV	Coefficient of variation
DOPA	Dihydroxyphenylalanin
EDTA	Ethylenediaminetetraacetic acid
EHC	Euglycaemic hyperinsulinemic clamp
ELISA	Enzyme-linked immunosorbent assay
EMS	Equine metabolic syndrome
FDR	False discovery rate
FIA	Flow injection analysis
FSIGTT	Frequently sampled intravenous glucose tolerance test
HDL	High-density lipoprotein
HI	Hyperinsulinemia
ID	Insulin dysregulation
IDO	Indoleamine 2,3-dioxygenase
IGF-1R	Insulin-like growth factor 1-receptor
IR	Insulin resistance
IST	Insulin stimulation test
LC	Liquid chromatography
LDL	Low-density lipoprotein
lysoPC	Lysophosphatidylcholine
MS/MS	Tandem mass spectrometry
NEFA	Non-esterified fatty acid
NMR	Nuclear magnetic resonance
OGT	Oral glucose test
PC	Phosphatidylcholine
PCR	Polymerase chain reaction

PLS-DA	Partial least-squares discriminant analysis
POMC	Pro-opiomelanocortin
PPID	Pituitary *pars intermedia* dysfunction
QC-RLSC	quality control-robust LOESS (locally estimated scatterplot smoothing) signal correction
$rAUC_{ins}$	Area under the insulin curve relatively to the mean area under the insulin curve of this individual
RPS6	Ribosomal protein S6
rWeight	Bodyweight relatively to the mean bodyweight of this horse
SGLT-2	Sodium-glucose co-transporter 2
SI	Insulin sensitivity
SM	Sphingomyelin
TCA	Tricarboxylic acid
VLDL	Very low-density lipoprotein

Summary

Julien Delarocque

Metabolic profiling of hyperinsulinemic horses

In horses, hyperinsulinemia occurs in association with insulin dysregulation, which comprises insulin resistance and basal or postprandial hyperinsulinemia. Insulin dysregulation plays a central role in equine endocrinopathies and mediates the increased risk for laminitis associated with these diseases. By describing the metabolic profile associated with insulin dysregulation, it was attempted to provide adjunct diagnostic tools for this condition but also to improve the understanding of its pathophysiology, with potential implications for therapy.

The data analysed in the present thesis originated from three distinct trials. First, three oral glucose tests were performed in twelve Icelandic horses. Their metabolic profile was described and put in relation to their level of insulin dysregulation (Manuscript 1). As expected, glucose influx and insulin effect lead to a decrease in proteolysis and enhanced cellular amino acid uptake. However, the kynurenine:tryptophan ratio increased during the test, possibly indicating low-grade inflammation. Additionally, carnitine, arginine and DOPA were significantly associated with the level of the insulin response, suggesting a potential involvement in pathological processes causing or resulting from insulin dysregulation. Beside the descriptive aspects, the predictive potential of the metabolite panel was investigated in a proof-of-concept approach. Encouraging results for the use of a restricted set of metabolites as biomarkers for insulin dysregulation were obtained.

Secondly, the bodyweight and metabolic profile of nineteen Icelandic horses were determined five times over one year, to (1) describe the development of their insulin response depending on the variations in bodyweight (Manuscript 2), and (2) to distinguish the impact of variations in bodyweight from the variations of the insulin response on the metabolome (Manuscript 3). It was found that a reduction of the bodyweight of 5% reduced the mean insulin response to the oral glucose test by over 20% and that these findings could be monitored with a simple two-time points oral glucose test. Moreover, an indicator of oxidative stress (trans-4-hydroxyproline) previously associated with insulin dysregulation itself, might rather be related to weight gain. The previously reported impact of insulin dysregulation on arginine metabolism was supported by indications of a higher arginase activity, while the hepatic metabolism might still be insulin sensitive despite insulin dysregulation.

Lastly, early samples from a high-sugar dietary challenge that triggered laminitis in some ponies but not in others were analysed on the metabolomic level to identify metabolic differences between laminitis-prone and -resistant ponies (Manuscript 4).

Again, potential indicators of hepatic insulin-sensitivity were present. On the other hand, the laminitis-prone ponies failed to show a reduction of their amino acid concentrations proportional to their insulin response, which is rather suggestive of a peripheral insulin resistance. The main differences between laminitis-prone and -resistant ponies were their phosphatidylcholine concentrations.

Altogether, these results provided new concepts for the identification of insulin dysregulation, supported an association between this condition and vascular dysfunction, helped distinguish the metabolic impact of weight variations from the effect of insulin dysregulation and suggested that carnitine and arginine could be investigated as nutritional supplements to treat insulin dysregulation.

Zusammenfassung

Julien Delarocque

Metabolisches Profil hyperinsulinämischer Pferde

Bei Pferden entsteht eine Hyperinsulinämie hauptsächlich im Zusammenhang mit einer Insulindysregulation, die Insulinresistenz und basale oder postprandiale Hyperinsulinämie umfasst. Diese Dysregulation ist als Bestandteil der wichtigsten endokrinologischen Erkrankungen des Pferdes von zentraler Bedeutung, da sie mit einem erhöhten Risiko für Hufrehe einhergeht. Die Beschreibung des metabolischen Profils betroffener Pferde sollte dazu dienen alternative diagnostische Möglichkeiten aufzuzeigen und das Verständnis der Pathophysiologie dieser Erkrankung zu erweitern.

Die in dieser These vorgestellten Daten sind im Rahmen von drei Versuchen entstanden. Zuerst wurden drei orale Glukosetests an zwölf Islandpferden durchgeführt und deren metabolisches Profil im Zusammenhang mit deren Insulinantwort untersucht (Manuskript 1). Wie erwartet kam es durch den Glukoseeinstrom und die Insulinsekretion zu einer Abnahme der Proteolyse und einer verstärkten Aufnahme von Aminosäuren durch die Zellen. Allerdings nahm auch das Kynurenin:Tryptophan-Verhältnis während des Tests zu, was als Hinweis auf eine unterschwellige Entzündung gewertet werden kann. Des Weiteren wurden starke Zusammenhänge zwischen Carnitin-, Arginin- und DOPA-Konzentrationenen und der Insulinantwort festgestellt, die auf pathologische Prozesse im Zusammenhang mit der Insulindysregulation hindeuten könnten. Nebst diesen deskriptiven Aspekten wurden die prädiktiven Eigenschaften des Metaboliten-Panels in einem Proof-of-Concept-Ansatz ermittelt. Dieser Ansatz lieferte Ergebnisse, die als Grundlage für die Entwicklung einer diagnostischen Plattform mit einer eingeschränkten Metabolitenanzahl dienen können.

In einem zweiten Untersuchungsteil wurden das Körpergewicht und metabolische Profile von neunzehn Islandpferden fünf Mal im Laufe eines Jahres ermittelt, um (1) die Entwicklung ihrer Insulinantwort im Zusammenhang mit Körpergewichtsschwankungen zu beschreiben (Manuskript 2) und (2) um den Einfluss der Körpergewichtsveränderungen auf das Metabolom von dem der Insulinantwort zu unterscheiden (Manuskript 3). Es wurde festgestellt, dass eine Gewichtsabnahme von 5% mit einem Rückgang der Insulinantwort um über 20% einherging und dass diese Entwicklung zuverlässig mit einem vereinfachten oralen Glukosetest mit zwei Messzeitpunkten zu kontrollieren war. Darüber hinaus wurde aus den Ergebnissen abgeleitet, dass das trans-4-Hydroxyprolin, ein Indikator für oxidativen Stress, eher mit Körpergewichtszunahmen als wie bisher vermutet mit der Insulindysregulation im

Zusammengang steht. Der zuvor beschriebene Einfluss einer Insulindysregulation auf den Arginin-Stoffwechsel wurde durch Hinweise auf eine erhöhte Arginase-Aktivität unterstützt, während der Lebermetabolismus trotz Insulindysregulation weiterhin insulinsensitiv erschien.

Zuletzt fand die metabolomische Auswertung von Proben statt, die im Rahmen eines Versuches zur Provokation von Hufrehe durch Fütterung einer zuckerhaltigen Diät entstanden waren (Manuskript 4). Das metabolische Profil ergab Hinweise auf einen insulinsensitiven Lebermetabolismus in beiden Kohorten. Andererseits zeigten die Hufrehe-empfindlichen Ponys unter Einfluss von Insulin keine vergleichbare Abnahme der Aminosäurenkonzentrationen, was eher für eine (möglicherweise periphere) Insulinresistenz spricht. Der Hauptunterschied zwischen den Hufrehe-empfindlichen und -resistenten Ponys bestand in abweichenden Phosphatidylcholinkonzentrationen.

Zusammenfassend ergaben sich aus diesen Ergebnissen neue Konzepte zur Diagnose der Insulindysregulation und Hinweise für eine Beeinträchtigung der Gefäßfunktion im Zusammenhang mit dieser Erkrankung. Die Untersuchungen zeigten, dass der Effekt von Gewichtsschwankungen auf das Metabolom von dem Effekt der Insulindysregulation auf das Metabolom unterschieden werden kann. Des Weiteren wurden neue Therapieansätze in Form einer Carnitin- und/oder Argininsupplementierung vorgeschlagen.

1. Introduction

The equine hoof consists of a horn capsule within which the distal phalanx is suspended to the heavily keratinized epidermis by outgrowths of the remarkably modified dermis called *laminae*. Thus, the weight of the animal is redirected towards the edge of the hoof wall facing the ground, while the sole is not bearing weight. Laminitis describes the failure of the attachment of the phalanx to the hoof wall and is often associated with pain and lameness [1].

The first written record of laminitis in history is commonly attributed to Xenophon (380 BC), describing a disease induced by barley surfeit [2]. Later authors also attributed laminitis to excessive grazing (grass founder) or strenuous work [2]. It is now recognized that laminitis can result from different kinds of primary diseases, such as sepsis or disruption of the gastro-intestinal barrier, or alimentary causes and excessive weight bearing, as described in early days. As a result, the research on laminitis made use of several models for laminitis induction. The widely used Obel grading system for laminitis was established using a sepsis model [3], while carbohydrate overload models became more predominant in the second half of the 20th century [2].

A possible endocrinological aetiology of laminitis was first put forward by Field and Jeffcott in 1986 [4], who linked the higher prevalence of this condition in obese ponies to their higher insulin response to an oral glucose test (OGT) compared to non-obese ponies and Standardbred horses. Retrospectively, these visionary experiments fit extraordinarily well with our current understanding of endocrinopathic laminitis. It took over twenty-five years for the term insulin dysregulation (ID), which describes the excessive insulin response to oral carbohydrates uncovered by Field and Jeffcott, to be coined [5]. Since endocrinopathic laminitis nowadays accounts for around 90% of laminitis cases [6], the underlying endocrinologic diseases have lately received considerable attention.

1.1. Equine hyperinsulinemia

Hyperinsulinemia (HI) describes an excessive insulin concentration in the blood. This can occur due to a reduced insulin clearance, as associated with insulin resistance (IR), and/or because of increased insulin secretion by the pancreatic β-cells. Pancreatic β-cell failure, as it occurs in type 2 diabetes mellitus, is very rare in horses and often associated with other diseases such as pancreatitis and endocrinologically active neoplasms [7]. Therefore, the pancreatic gland can sustain an increased insulin production for a long time, as compared to humans [8].

The term ID encompasses basal HI, IR and (transient) postprandial HI resulting from an excessive insulin response to an oral glucose stimulus. The latter was hypothesized to result from incretin stimulation, although differences in incretin concentrations in healthy and dysregulated horses could not be detected consistently [9,10]. Regardless of its underlying cause, ID results in HI at one time or another.

Since insulin secretion is part of a complex, dynamic equilibrium between energy carriers in different compartments and multidirectional hormonal control mechanisms, there is no single cut-off defining HI. The diagnostic tests for ID will be discussed later. In general, cut-offs have been established by describing the insulin response to certain test protocols in healthy and diseased cohorts, as defined by another reference test or other factors such as obesity or predisposition for laminitis [11,12]. More recently, efforts have been made to distinguish healthy and diseased animals in a less arbitrary, multivariate, clustering-based approach [13]. However, ID is neither due do congenital disorders of the metabolism (even if genetic factors can contribute to its development), nor a fundamentally irreversible state, since sufficient weight loss may normalize the insulin response of affected horses [14]. Therefore, it appears more likely that this condition can be present in different gradual intensities than that it can be described using timepoint-specific dichotomous cut-offs. As a result, the total insulin response to defined stimuli (mathematically described by the area under the insulin curve during a dynamic test) has been used as continuous measure of ID [15–19]. Nevertheless, cut-offs remain valuable in a practical setting, where it must be decided if an intervention is required or not. To add to the confusion, there are notable discrepancies between different insulin assays [20–25], so that cut-offs must be considered assay specific. All in all, the definition of HI is context dependent.

The equine metabolic syndrome (EMS) describes a range of risk factors for endocrinopathic laminitis. The term was first introduced by Johnson in 2002 [26] and its definition later clarified in two successive consensus statements [27,28]. The key feature of EMS is ID. Generalized or regional adiposity and a predisposition to weight gain are generally present and can be accompanied by secondary metabolic disorders such as hypertriglyceridemia, hypoadiponectinemia, hyperleptinemia and cardiovascular changes [28].

Another major endocrinologic disease of the horse is pituitary *pars intermedia* dysfunction (PPID). It is a neurodegenerative disorder resulting from the loss of dopaminergic inhibition of the pituitary *pars intermedia*, thus quantitatively and qualitatively altering the secretory activity of the pituitary gland. The clinical signs include hypertrichosis, muscle atrophy, polyuria and polydipsia, hyperhidrosis and abnormal fat distribution [29]. In addition, many affected horses suffer from ID, putting them a risk for laminitis. While the mechanisms causing ID in horses with PPID are not yet fully elucidated, they might differ from the ones prevailing in horses with EMS [5]. Indeed, IR appears to play a more prominent role in PPID than in EMS, because PPID affects the peripheral glucocorticoid metabolism [30].

To summarize, PPID and EMS are the two major endocrinopathies in equids. While ID is an essential part of EMS, not all horses with PPID suffer from ID. Nevertheless, both diseases are associated with an increased risk of laminitis, which is conveyed by ID and the resulting HI. There is little epidemiological data regarding the prevalence of EMS, but the prevalence of HI was reported to be around 27% in ponies [31] and 20% in horses [32,33]. Obesity is a major risk factor for both EMS and ID and was found in approximately 20–30% of horses with seasonal variations [34,35]. In contrast, 2.9% of equids were affected by PPID in a systematic review, but this proportion increased to 21.2% in horses and ponies aged over 15 years [36].

Hyperinsulinemia can also occur in conditions promoting IR or hyperglycaemia, such as systemic infection and inflammation or gestation and hormonally active neoplasms. However, such cases will not be discussed in the present work.

1.2. Insulin-associated laminitis

Laminitis reportedly affects around 3% of equids all causes included, but the reported estimates vary greatly depending on the study population [37]. It should be stressed that this disease is painful and can require euthanasia in severe cases. The most frequent aetiology of laminitis is highlighted in the terms 'endocrinopathic laminitis' and 'insulin-associated laminitis'. The denomination 'grass founder' describes a chronic form of 'pasture-associated laminitis', which occurs in predisposed horses because of the insulin response engendered by grazing on lush pasture. The causal link between HI and laminitis was experimentally demonstrated [38–40] and is supported by the description of insulinaemia in laminitis-prone animals as compared to healthy ones [41–46].

The (human) metabolic syndrome is defined as a collection of risk factors for cardiovascular disease and type 2 diabetes mellitus [47]. While IR plays a more prominent role in humans than in horses, it is considered that HI is the initial cause of the clinical manifestations of the metabolic syndrome [48], legitimizing the term EMS. The (hypothesized) mechanisms by which HI induces IR, hypertension, dyslipidaemia, and inflammation are as manifold as the metabolic processes involving insulin. While some of these mechanisms might be transposable to equids, a mechanistic explanation of the relationship between HI and laminitis is still lacking. The previously investigated hypotheses of glucotoxicity [49] and glucose deprivation within the *laminae* [50] have been rejected. There is evidence of some forms of vascular dysfunction occurring in laminitic horses and a model of vascular IR [51,52]; however, the potential impact on the lamellar epithelial cells remains unclear. Recently, the insulin-like growth factor-1 receptor (IGF-1R) and a hybrid insulin/ IGF-1R have been highlighted as potential binding targets for insulin in the lamellar tissue during HI [53,54]. These receptors are involved in the regulation of cell growth, adhesion, proliferation, differentiation and apoptosis [54]. The ribosomal protein S6 (RPS6) is activated by IGF-1R and regulates actin remodelling. Therefore, it could be involved in the elongation of epithelial cells, which is a major feature of lamellar histopathology in endocrinopathic laminitis [53].

1.3. Metabolic profile associated with insulin dysregulation

By definition, EMS is associated with ID, which can manifest as IR but also as permanent or transient HI. While IR is said to often occur secondarily to HI, insulin sensitive hyperinsulinemic phenotypes exist as well [10,55]. This phenotypic heterogeneity even in the most fundamental aspect of EMS explains why further metabolic dysregulations can be very variable amongst affected individuals. Likewise, EMS is often associated with obesity, but the existence of a lean EMS phenotype was also demonstrated [56,57]. As summarized in **Figure 1**, the different aspects of ID are interrelated.

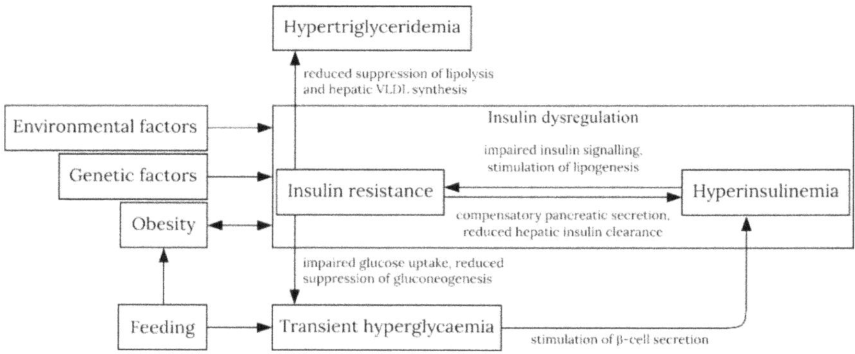

Figure 1 Graphical summary of the relationship between different aspects of EMS and their metabolic impact. VLDL: very low-density lipoprotein. Partly based on [28].

1.3.1. Previously described alterations of the metabolism

Hypertriglyceridemia is sometimes present in ID and EMS [41,56,58]. Besides triglycerides, increased non-esterified fatty acid (NEFA) [58], high-density lipoprotein (HDL) and low-density lipoprotein (LDL) cholesterol concentrations were also reported by some authors [58,59]. Nevertheless, most lipid fractions did not consistently differ between obese IR and IS [60,61], so that dyslipidaemia might rather be associated with further variables like the genotype, feeding, severity of obesity, etc. [61]. Hormonal differences include hyperleptinemia [58,62] and hypoadiponectinemia [63–65]. The connection between these hormones and obesity [66] nicely illustrates that it is difficult to isolate the effect of HI on the metabolism from its confounders. Such problems are also encountered when studying animals with concurrent PPID and ID, where an altered glucocorticoid metabolism might contribute to the development of peripheral IR [30].

Inflammation and oxidative stress have long been suspected to play a role in ID and laminitis [67]. However, while some mediators of inflammation such as interleukin 1 (IL-1) and tumour necrosis factor α (TNF-α) [68] appear to be associated with IR, the pathways activated by these conditions appear to be rather specific and it is difficult to support the hypothesis of a generalized (pro-)inflammatory state [69]. Nevertheless, the protracted inflammatory response to endotoxins observed in horses with EMS [70] might suggest that this condition impairs the dynamic response to certain stimuli, rather than it affects basal indicators of inflammation. In the same way, the antioxidative capacities of muscle tissue were positively correlated with the body condition score (BCS) but there was no evidence of oxidative damage [42]. Still, the available evidence regarding oxidative damage in these conditions remains contradictory [33,49,71].

1.3.2. Technical aspects

The phenotypic characterization of ID can take place on different levels. While hormone and other peptide concentrations are often determined with immunoassays [20,25,72–75], polymerase chain reaction (PCR) was mainly used to quantify gene expression [76–81]. However, the individual measurement of more broad sets of molecules can become tedious. When exploring metabolites associated with energy metabolism, high-throughput approaches relying on nuclear magnetic resonance (NMR) or mass spectrometry in combination with chromatographic techniques have become increasingly popular in both humans and livestock [82,83]. The identification of biomolecules can take place in a targeted or untargeted fashion, requiring different levels of expertise and effort (untargeted approaches being more complicated). The large range of small molecules present in an organ or organism is called metabolome and their large-scale estimation is called metabolomics. Such approaches have been employed to describe the metabolome of horses and ponies during OGT [84,85], lamellar tissue bioenergetics in an oligofructose laminitis model [86] and impact of obesity on the metabolome in horses [87]. Interesting results include an impairment of the tricarboxylic acid (TCA) cycle in insulin-dysregulated ponies [85], increase of circulating free fatty acids in obese horses [87] and signs of pro-inflammatory events during the OGT [84].

1.4. Diagnosing insulin dysregulation

Because of its implications for animal welfare, the early identification of ID is crucial. The identification of risk factors for laminitis or ID is not obvious to most horse owners [88,89] and should be communicated by the veterinarian. Testing should be considered when signs of metabolic disease become obvious (see above), significant weight gain is observed or when there is a history of laminitis [28].

Several methods for quantification of insulin have been in use in equids in recent years but did not provide perfect agreement nor a linear relationship [20–25], so that reference ranges and cut-off values should be considered assay-specific. Additionally, it is agreed that higher insulin concentrations are associated with a higher risk of laminitis. Therefore, as mentioned previously, the use of cut-off values is not necessarily the best representation of the spectrum of ID [13].

1.4.1. Basal testing

As mentioned earlier, ID encompasses basal HI, IR, and postprandial HI. Therefore, the simplest way to diagnose ID is to measure insulin in a fasted animal. An insulin concentration in blood lower than 20 µIU/ml is typically considered to rule out basal hyperinsulinemia [90]. Nevertheless, many dysregulated horses have inconspicuous basal insulin values so that the exclusion of ID based on such results is likely to be impaired by false negative errors [28].

Fasting blood glucose concentration is of little use in horses with ID, because they usually manage to maintain normoglycemia (when solely affected by ID) [12]. Hyperglycaemia is rather considered indicative of type 2 diabetes mellitus. The combination of basal glucose and insulin concentrations in ratios and proxies was found to correlate with tests for IR and might be more useful than basal glucose or insulin alone [91,92].

The use of biomarkers other than insulin and glucose (ideally in basal samples to avoid tiresome testing) has also been investigated. For example, adiponectin was reported to have 80% sensitivity and specificity to predict pasture-associated laminitis in the next three years [46] although it correlated poorly with insulin [12]. On the other hand, it remains that insulin is per definition the most sensitive indicator of ID.

1.4.2. Detecting insulin resistance

Owing to its most prominent role in human endocrinology, there are plentiful tests for the diagnosis of IR. Generally, these tests rely on the intravenous administration of glucose, insulin, or both in a predetermined dosage. The most complex of these tests is the euglycemic hyperinsulinemic clamp (EHC) [93,94], which allows to quantify several aspects of insulin and glucose dynamics using the insulin and glucose infusion rate and is considered the gold standard. Simpler, but still laborious protocols are the frequently sampled intravenous glucose tolerance test (FSIGTT) [95] and combined glucose insulin tolerance test (CGIT) [96]. These protocols basically use glucose and insulin boluses instead of constant rate infusions to achieve similar results to the EHC. Lastly, the insulin stimulation test (IST) depends on the simple assumption that an insulin bolus should be followed by a timely reduction of the blood glucose concentration [97]. A comparatively short protocol (30 min) and a good repeatability make this test suitable for clinical use. However, the amount of information it delivers is more limited.

1.4.3. The advantages of oral testing protocols

Oral test protocols (such as the previously mentioned OGT used by Field and Jeffcott [4]) measure the insulin response to an oral glucose stimulation. The way of application and dosage of glucose (or glycaemic preparation) may vary [12,28]. While these tests are subject to greater within individual variation [12], they are more similar to naturally occurring stimuli [9,28]. The differences in the results yielded by tests of IR and oral tests arise from the fact that firstly, not all horses with ID are insulin-resistant, and secondly, glucose-related enteric mechanisms appear to play a role in ID. Consequently, oral tests are currently the recommended method for the diagnosis of ID [28].

1.5. Treating insulin dysregulation

1.5.1. Current recommendations

Since the positive correlation between obesity or weight gain and measures of IR has long been established [4], weight loss programs have been investigated early on as a possible therapy and proven rather effective [15,81,98–100]. As a result, the main recommendation for the treatment of EMS is to promote weight loss [28]. Many dietary protocols have been suggested and generally relied on the exclusion of cereal-based components and restriction of the roughage to a certain percentage of the (optimal) bodyweight [101]. It is acknowledged that some horses appear to be weight loss resistant and require even more drastic measures [14].

The concurrent promotion of exercise was often found useful [81,98,99] and some authors even reported that dietary restrictions alone were ineffective [98] – a question on which there is also no agreement in human medicine [102,103]. It could be argued that this effect relies on the endocrine activity of the musculoskeletal system which even affects adipocyte growth [104,105]. Additionally, a punctual intensive mobilization of energy storages during exercise is likely to affect their responsiveness. Nevertheless, besides methodological differences among these experiments (e.g., energy content and source, exercise intensity and duration), there are numerous confounders which might have influenced the results (age, sex, genetic background, season, initial severity of IR to name a few). Owing to these limitations, it is also difficult to quantify the amount of weight loss required to reduce the insulin response and it remains unknown if similar results can be achieved independently of the initial bodyweight (i.e., proportionality and linearity). Lastly, most of these experiments have used measures of IR and not of ID, ignoring the enteric component of EMS [10], which might not be affected by these measures in the same way.

1.5.2. Pharmacological treatment

The pharmacological treatment of ID should not be used as a primary therapy but rather as an adjunctive one in cases refractory to weight loss [28]. Three major alternatives have been explored (1) sensitization to insulin, (2) reduction of glucose availability, and (3) increase of the metabolic rate.

The insulin-sensitizer pioglitazone is used in type 2 diabetes mellitus in humans but failed to improve IS in horses [106]. Metformin is also known as insulin-sensitizer in humans but apparently fails to reach satisfying concentrations in horses because of poor bioavailability [107]. Nevertheless, it was able to reduce estimates of IR in several trials, which was partly attributed to its effect on enterocytes [108–111]. Recently, the sodium-glucose co-transporter 2 (SGLT-2) inhibitor velagliflozin, which induces glucose loss through the renal excretion, was shown to improve HI and prevent laminitis in a preliminary trial [112]. Lastly, levothyroxine treatment helped in reducing body mass by increasing the metabolic rate and insulin sensitivity (SI) [113].

1.6. Hypotheses (H), aims (A) and objectives (O)

Insulin is responsible for the distribution of carbohydrates, fats, and further essential molecules throughout the body. Its synthesis and release are regulated by the availability of these substrates, while its effects include the synthesis of energy-carriers and proteins. Given its central role in metabolism and key position in ID, the primary hypothesis of the present thesis was that

(H1) *ID is associated with fundamental changes of the metabolome.*

To (A1.1) derive biomarkers of ID from the metabolic profile, (O1.1) the metabolic profile of horses with and without ID was compared in a basal state and during an induced hyperinsulinemia. Additionally, it was sought to (A1.2) identify pathological changes of the metabolome associated with ID by (O1.2) correlating the metabolic profile with the level of ID.

Obesity is a major risk factor for ID and weight loss is consequently the major aim of the therapy for this condition. However, previous work on the impact of obesity on

ID was primarily focused on IR and did not describe the relationship between both parameters to its full extent. As a result, it was hypothesized that

(H2) *weight loss leads to a proportional reduction of the level of ID.*

To (A2) describe the relationship between weight variations and the level of ID, (O2) the changes of the insulin response to the OGT was analysed depending on the concurrent changes in body weight.

Having addressed the relationship between ID and weight variations, it appeared important to relate these findings to the previously assessed metabolic impact of ID. As there are obese normoinsulinemic and lean insulin resistant individuals, the hypothesis that

(H3) *weight gain and aggravation of ID have a distinct impact on the metabolome*

was formulated. (A3) The concurrent description of the impact of weight gain and the fluctuations of ID on the metabolome, was achieved (O3) by correlating the metabolic profile of horses with the development of their body weight and insulin response over time during repeated OGTs.

It was then aimed to transfer the previously addressed topics to the main clinical manifestation of ID. Because insulin plays a central role in the metabolism but is also central in the pathophysiology of endocrinopathic laminitis, it was hypothesized that

(H4) *the development of laminitis can be predicted by the metabolic profile.*

Therefore, it was attempted to (A4) identify biomarkers of subsequent laminitis development by (O4) comparing the metabolome of laminitis-resistant and laminitis-prone ponies.

Since endocrinopathic laminitis is mostly associated with long-standing metabolic dysregulation and/or obesity, it was finally investigated whether

(H5) *the subsequent development of laminitis is primed by pre-existent metabolic changes.*

To (A5) identify metabolic differences associated with subsequent laminitis, (O5) the basal metabolome and metabolic response to a high-sugar diet of laminitis-resistant and laminitis-prone ponies were compared.

2. Manuscript 1

Metabolic changes induced by oral glucose tests in horses and their diagnostic use

Julien Delarocque[1]*, Florian Frers[1], Karsten Feige[1], Korinna Huber[2], Klaus Jung[3], Tobias Warnken[1]

[1] Clinic for Horses, University of Veterinary Medicine Hannover, Foundation, Hannover, Germany.

[2] Institute of Animal Science, Faculty of Agricultural Sciences, University of Hohenheim, Stuttgart, Germany.

[3] Institute for Animal Breeding and Genetics, University of Veterinary Medicine Hannover, Foundation, Hannover, Germany.

* Corresponding author

State of publication:

Published in Journal of Veterinary Internal Medicine (2020) 1–9
DOI: 10.1111/jvim.15992

Contributions to the manuscript:

T. Warnken and K. Feige designed the experiments. J. Delarocque and F. Frers performed the experiments. J. Delarocque measured the insulin concentrations, prepared the figures, and wrote the paper. J. Delarocque and K. Jung analysed the data. All authors contributed to the interpretation of the results, reviewed drafts of the paper, and accepted the final manuscript.

Received: 14 April 2020 | Accepted: 20 November 2020
DOI: 10.1111/jvim.15992

STANDARD ARTICLE

Journal of Veterinary Internal Medicine Open Access

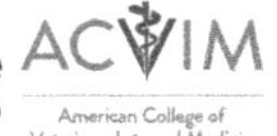

Metabolic changes induced by oral glucose tests in horses and their diagnostic use

Julien Delarocque[1] | Florian Frers[1] | Karsten Feige[1] | Korinna Huber[2] | Klaus Jung[3] | Tobias Warnken[1]

[1]Clinic for Horses, University of Veterinary Medicine Hannover, Foundation, Hanover, Germany

[2]Institute of Animal Science, Faculty of Agricultural Sciences, University of Hohenheim, Stuttgart, Germany

[3]Institute for Animal Breeding and Genetics, University of Veterinary Medicine Hannover, Foundation, Hanover, Germany

Correspondence
Julien Delarocque, Clinic for Horses, University of Veterinary Medicine Hannover, Foundation, Bünteweg 9, 30559, Hanover, Germany.
Email: julien.delarocque@tiho-hannover.de

Abstract

Background: Little is known about the implications of hyperinsulinemia on energy metabolism, and such knowledge might help understand the pathophysiology of insulin dysregulation.

Objectives: Describe differences in the metabolic response to an oral glucose test, depending on the magnitude of the insulin response.

Animals: Twelve Icelandic horses in various metabolic states.

Methods: Horses were subjected to 3 oral glucose tests (OGT; 0.5 g/kg body weight glucose). Basal, 120 and 180 minutes samples were analyzed using a combined liquid chromatography tandem mass spectrometry and flow injection analysis tandem mass spectrometry metabolomic assay. Insulin concentrations were measured using an ELISA. Analysis was performed using linear models and partial least-squares regression.

Results: The kynurenine : tryptophan ratio increased over time during the OGT (adjusted *P*-value = .001). A high insulin response was associated with lower arginine (adjusted *P*-value = .02) and carnitine (adjusted *P*-value = .03) concentrations. A predictive model using only baseline samples performed well with as few as 7 distinct metabolites (sensitivity, 86%; 95% confidence interval [CI], 81%-90%; specificity, 88%; 95% CI, 84%-92%).

Conclusions and Clinical Importance: Our results suggest induction of low-grade inflammation during the OGT. Plasma arginine and carnitine concentrations were lower in horses with high insulin response and could constitute potential therapeutic targets. Development of screening tools to identify insulin-dysregulated horses using only baseline blood sample appears promising.

KEYWORDS
biomarker, EMS, insulin dysregulation, metabolomics, oral glucose test

Abbreviations: AUC_{ins}, area under the insulin curve over time; EMS, equine metabolic syndrome; HI, hyperinsulinemia; ID, insulin dysregulation; LysoPC, lysophosphatidylcholine; NPV, negative predictive value; OGT, oral glucose test; PC, phosphatidylcholine; PLS-DA, partial least-squares discriminant analysis; PPV, positive predictive value; SM, sphingomyelin.

1 | INTRODUCTION

Equine metabolic syndrome (EMS) encompasses a range of disorders of energy metabolism, bearing some similarities with metabolic syndrome as defined in humans.[1] Insulin dysregulation (ID), including insulin resistance and transient or long lasting hyperinsulinemia (HI),[2] and regional or generalized adiposity are seen as major risk factors for laminitis,[3] which is central to the definition of EMS. This disorder of the dermoepidermal attachment within the hoof in fact can be directly induced by HI, either experimentally[4,5] or as a result of an exaggerated pancreatic insulin secretion in response to PO carbohydrate intake,[6] but also might be promoted by proinflammatory factors observed in ID or EMS patients.[7-9]

The oral glucose test (OGT) consists of administration of a fixed amount of glucose via nasogastric tube. By subsequently measuring insulin concentrations in blood, the insulin response can be quantified, providing a diagnostic tool for identification of HI[10] and prediction of laminitis risk.[6] Furthermore, the insulin response to the OGT appears to be correlated with the insulin response to grazing.[11]

Many studies have been undertaken to identify markers of the inflammatory processes associated with HI, laminitis, or obesity in horses.[12-15] By using a metabolomics approach, cellular processes of this kind can be identified. The mechanisms triggered by carbohydrate intake during the OGT are of interest, because they might reflect what happens when hyperinsulinemic horses are grazing. Analysis of baseline samples could identify long sought biomarkers of HI useful for diagnostic screening and limit the requirement for OGT and other complex tests.

As a result, our aim was to investigate the impact of the OGT on the metabolome in healthy and hyperinsulinemic horses. Metabolites involved in inflammatory processes or linked to metabolic diseases were targeted. In contrast to previous studies of the metabolomic response of horses to the OGT,[16,17] the area under the curve of insulin over time (AUC_{Ins}) was used as a continuous predictor in a linear model, allowing for a more detailed description of the relationship between the insulin response and the metabolome. Additionally, the performance of predictive models was explored to investigate the discriminatory potential of the candidate biomarkers.

2 | MATERIALS AND METHODS

2.1 | Horses

Twelve Icelandic horses (5 geldings and 7 mares) aged 9 to 29 years (median, 19 years) were enrolled in the study. They were fed hay ad libitum and kept in barns and paddocks. Access to pasture was allowed every day for up to 6 hours. A full clinical examination and thyrotropin releasing hormone stimulation test were performed after the standard protocol[18] and before the beginning of the experiments to rule out clinical disorders other than ID. The State Office for Consumer Protection and Food Safety (LAVES) approved the study in accordance with the German Animal Welfare Law (file number: 33.19-42 502-05-17A099).

2.2 | Oral glucose tests

Three OGTs were performed over a period of 7 weeks with 3- and 4-week intervals between the first and second, and second and third OGT, respectively. The horses were fasted overnight before testing. The next morning an indwelling catheter (Intraflon 2 12 G, Vygon, Ecouen, France) was placed in a jugular vein for blood sample collection. After collection of a basal blood sample, 0.5 g/kg body weight glucose (Glucose, WDT, Garbsen, Germany) dissolved in 2 L of water was administered via a nasogastric tube. Additional blood samples were taken at 30, 60, 120, 180, and 240 minutes. All samples were collected into potassium EDTA and Z serum clot activator vacuum tubes (Vacuette, greiner bio-one, Kremsmünster, Austria). The EDTA tubes were chilled at 4°C and the serum tubes were allowed to clot at room temperature. They were centrifuged at 4000*g* for 10 minutes within 6 hours of collection, and the plasma and serum supernatants collected, aliquoted, and stored at −80°C.

2.3 | Insulin measurement

Serum insulin concentrations from all samples were measured in duplicate using a previously validated[19] equine insulin ELISA (Mercodia Equine Insulin ELISA, Mercodia AB, Uppsala, Sweden; interassay coefficient of variation, 7.7%) following manufacturer's instructions. When insulin concentration exceeded the range of quantification, serum samples were diluted 1:4 using diabetes sample buffer (Mercodia Diabetes Sample Buffer, Mercodia AB).

2.4 | Metabolomic assay

Metabolic profiling of basal, 120 and 180 minutes EDTA plasma samples was performed using the Biocrates AbsoluteIDQ p180 Kit (Biocrates Life Sciences AG, Innsbruck, Austria). This assay includes up to 188 metabolites related to glycolysis, oxidative processes, lipid degradation, and inflammatory signaling. For example, acylcarnitines are related to fatty acid oxidation and fatty acid profiles[20] whereas the phospholipids (phosphatidylcholines [PCs], lysophosphatidylcholines [LysoPCs], and sphingomyelins [SMs]), which are major components of lipid membranes, also are involved in cell signaling.[21] Many such molecules previously have been linked to insulin action[22] or metabolic conditions in several species.[9,20,23,24] The total length of the fatty acid chains, number of double bonds, and bond types are indicated in the molecule annotation. For example, PC aa C34:3 represents PC, the 2 fatty acids of which are bound to glycerol via ester bonds (aa, acyl-acyl; ae, acyl-alkyl). Its 2 fatty acids have a combined length of 34 C atoms and 3 double bonds. Because acylcarnitines, hexoses, PC, LysoPC, and SMs were quantified using flow injection analysis-tandem mass spectrometry, the lipid species can correspond to several isomers. In contrast, amino acids, and biogenic amines were measured by liquid chromatography-tandem mass spectrometry. These measurements were performed at the Fraunhofer Institute of Toxicology and Experimental Medicine ITEM, Hanover, Germany.

2.5 | Statistical analysis

The methods used for statistical analysis are described in detail in supplementary file 1. Briefly, metabolites that did not pass quality control were removed. Data were adjusted for batch effects, $\log_2$-tranformed, scaled, and quantile normalized.[25]

Linear models, as implemented in the "limma" R-package,50 were used to identify metabolites significantly associated with time in the OGT and AUC_{ins}. *P*-values were adjusted for multiple comparisons using the procedure of Benjamini and Hochberg.[26]

Partial least-squares discriminant analyses (PLS-DA) were conducted using the "DiscriMiner" R-package[27] to identify the most important metabolites for classification of horses depending on their total insulin response (2 arbitrarily defined, equally sized groups with either high or low AUC_{ins}). This analysis was performed separately for the basal and 120 minutes time point.

Metabolite importance was quantified using the variable importance in projection (VIP) score. This score can be interpreted as an indicator of the diagnostic value of the individual metabolites. Metabolites strongly correlated with HI and displaying a good separation between both groups generally are associated with higher VIP scores. To compare theses scores across models, they were scaled to a percentage value of the max VIP score within each model. As a result, the most important variable in each model was attributed a scaled VIP score of 100%.

Lastly, PLS-DA was repeated on the baseline dataset while varying the number of metabolites included in the model as a hyperparameter during a bootstrap cross-validation. Metabolites were removed by order of increasing importance as determined in the full model. Model performance (accuracy, sensitivity, specificity, positive predictive value [PPV], and negative predictive value [NPV]) was estimated using holdout data. These estimates were adjusted for the mean reported prevalence of HI.[28-30] The aim of this second approach was to determine the accuracy of smaller metabolite sets as predictors of HI in basal samples.

3 | RESULTS

One horse was diagnosed with pituitary pars intermedia dysfunction (PPID). No treatment was initiated before the end of the trials.

3.1 | Data preparation

The Biocrates AbsoluteIDQ p180 Kit measures plasma concentrations of up to 188 metabolites belonging to 6 substance classes. By summarizing these classes and adding the kynurenine : tryptophan ratio, 194 features are obtained. Data preprocessing decreased this number to 145, as detailed in Table 1. Twelve horses were subjected to 3 OGTs for each of which the time points 0, 120 and 180 minutes were considered in the metabolome, resulting in 108 samples. These time points were selected because of cost constraints to include baseline, insulin peak, and standard diagnostic time points. No outliers were found using the "bagplot" method.

TABLE 1 Metabolites available before and after data preprocessing. Summarized values are the sums of plasma concentrations of metabolites by groups (eg, sum of acylcarnitines) or ratios such as the kynurenine : tryptohphan ratio, which is of interest in the scope of inflammatory processes

Metabolite class	Before preprocessing	After preprocessing
Acylcarnitines	40	7
Amino acids	21	21
Biogenic amines	21	20
Glycerophospholipids	90	75
Sphingolipids	15	15
Sugars	1	1
Summarized values	6	6
Sum	194	145

3.2 | Linear model

Figure 1A graphically displays the progression of the significant features sorted by class. The sum of hexoses (H1) and dihydroxyphenylalanine (DOPA) increased upon glucose administration. Of all amino acids, only glycine (Gly) and tryptophan (Trp) increased over time whereas the others decreased. Similarly, among the glycerophospholipids, LysoPCs decreased whereas PCs increased, and except for the increasing carnitine (C0) and propionylcarnitine (C3), all acylcarnitines decreased.

The patterns associated with AUC_{ins} were less clear . All differentially concentrated acylcarnitines but also arginine (Arg) and spermidine were negatively associated with AUC_{ins}, in contrast to the only represented glycerophospholipid (PC ae C38:6), which was found in higher concentrations in horses with high insulin response (Figure 1B).

3.3 | Variable importance in PLS-DA

Indicators of model performance for both the baseline and 120 minutes model are summarized in Table 2. Overall, similar values were observed, but the baseline model appeared to be slightly more specific.

Figure 2 displays the scaled VIP scores for both models. Acetylcarnitine (C2) and the sum of acylcarnitines appear to be among the most important predictors for a high insulin response both at

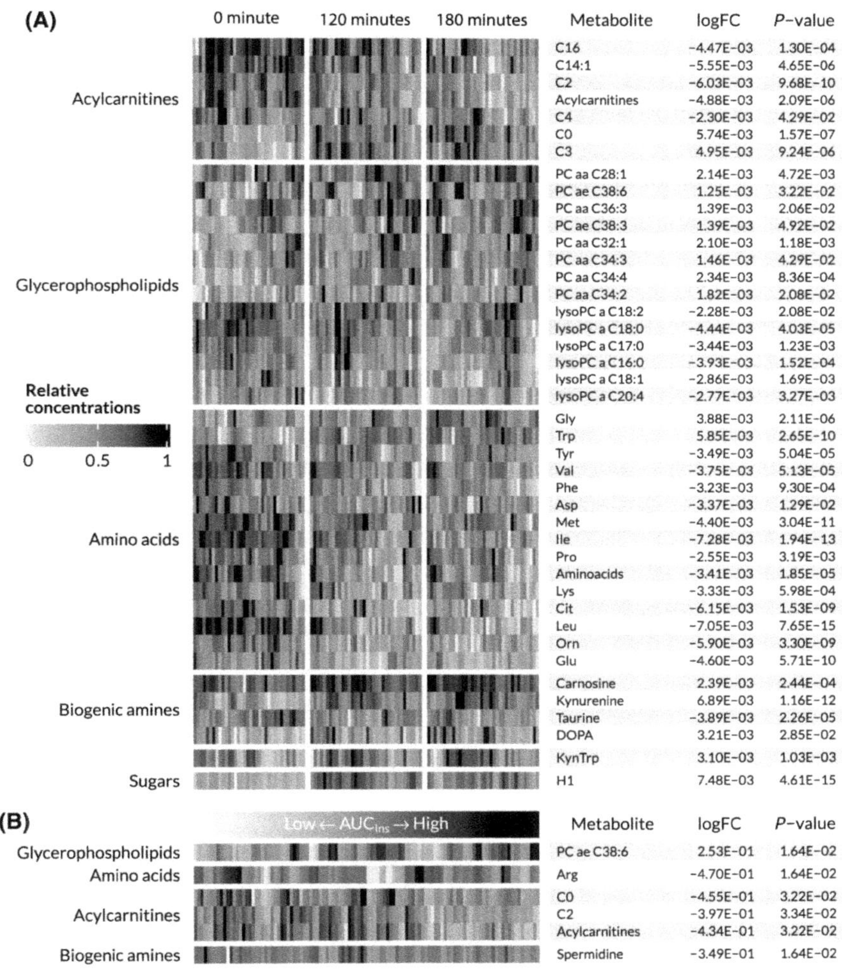

FIGURE 1 Heatmap of the relative metabolite concentrations for the metabolites significantly associated with (A) time during the oral glucose test (OGT) and (B) area under the insulin curve over time (AUC_{ins}). Each column of the heatmap represents a sample and each row a metabolite. In A, the samples are grouped by time point, whereas in B they are ordered by AUC_{ins} in ascending order. Metabolite names are displayed on the right side with associated fold change and adjusted P-values. In the case of numeric predictors like "Time" or "AUC_{ins}," the $\log_2$ fold change (logFC) given by the "limma" package represents the slope of the regression line. For each unit of the predictor (eg, time in minutes), the $\log_2$-transformed normalized metabolite concentrations thus increase by $\log_2$ FC. Note that all lysophosphatidylcholines decreased over time—as on average the colored tiles are darker at 0 than 180 minutes—whereas phosphatidylcholines increased. The associations between metabolites and AUC_{ins} were less apparent, because there was more individual variability

baseline and 120 minutes after glucose intake. In contrast, although still among the most important metabolites, some molecules such as symmetric (SDMA) and asymmetric (ADMA) dimethylarginine or alanine (Ala) had more variation in their associated VIP scores, indicating that their discriminatory potential differs more clearly between the baseline and 120 minutes models.

3.4 | Performance of reduced PLS-DA models on baseline samples

To investigate if identification of horses with high AUC_{ins} also was possible with fewer metabolites, the baseline PLS-DA model was rerun repeatedly with fewer and fewer metabolites in a bootstrap approach. Model performance for each of these repetitions is presented in Figure 3. The metabolites included in each run can be derived from the VIP scores in the full baseline PLS-DA model provided as supplemental Table S1. Because a bootstrap approach with more validation samples was used in comparison to the leave-one-out cross-validation used beforehand (see variable importance in PLS-DA), the overfitting often present in PLS-DA models with more features than samples resulted in a loss of performance when more metabolites were used, because fewer samples were available to train the model. Overall, model performance increased when decreasing the number of predictors. Specificity and PPV were maximized at 7, accuracy at 30, and sensitivity and NPV at 59 metabolites. With as few as 2 metabolites, accuracy, sensitivity, and NPV were within their respective 5 highest values.

TABLE 2 Indicators of model performance for the baseline and 120 minutes partial least-squares discriminant analysis (PLS-DA) as obtained by leave-one-out-cross-validation on all samples. Positive and negative predictive values were calculated using a prevalence of 22.5%

Parameter	Baseline	120 minutes
Accuracy	83% (67%-94%)	83% (67%-94%)
Sensitivity	78% (52%-94%)	83% (59%-96%)
Specificity	89% (65%-99%)	83% (59%-96%)
Positive predictive value	68% (32%-93%)	60% (28%-86%)
Negative predictive value	93% (76%-99%)	94% (77%-100%)

4 | DISCUSSION

Our objective was to investigate the metabolic response of horses during the OGT with a targeted metabolomics approach. The time course of metabolite concentrations and their relationship to the total insulin response, approximated as AUC_{ins}, were analyzed and the predictive power of the metabolite set was explored.

4.1 | Effects attributable to insulin action

The time course of metabolite concentrations during the OGT (Figure 1A) was linked to the pharmacokinetics and pharmacodynamics of glucose intake and insulin secretion. Because of the high glucose influx, the sum of hexoses (H1) is roughly equivalent to the glucose concentration during the OGT. Unsurprisingly, an increase in glucose can be observed over time, with a slight decrease from 120 to 180 minutes. The fold change of H1 can be used as a scale to interpret the shifts in other metabolites, because it should have the highest magnitude.

Of the 14 amino acids that varied significantly over time, only Trp and Gly had a positive concentration gradient during the test, whereas all others were negative. The decrease in amino acids corroborates previous reports on the metabolome during the OGT in humans and horses and could be attributed to insulin-induced decreased proteolysis and enhanced cellular amino acid uptake.[9,31,32]

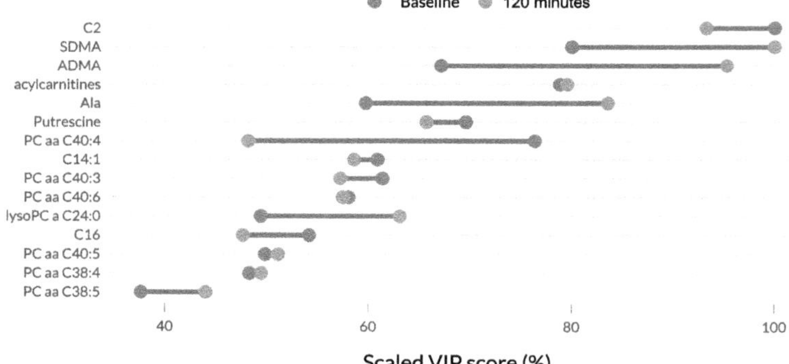

FIGURE 2 Dumbbell plot of the scaled Variable Importance in Projection (VIP) scores of the top 10 metabolites from the baseline and 120 minutes partial least-squares discriminant analysis (PLS-DA) models. The scaling of the scores allows for a better comparability between models. As there is some overlap between the 10 metabolites in each model, the combination of both rankings results in the 15 metabolites displayed here. The dark segments between pairs of points represent the difference in relative importance of the metabolites. Large differences indicate that although the metabolite is very helpful in distinguishing horses with a high area under the insulin curve over time (AUC_{ins}) from horses with a low 1in- model, the difference between both groups regarding this metabolite is less striking at the other time point

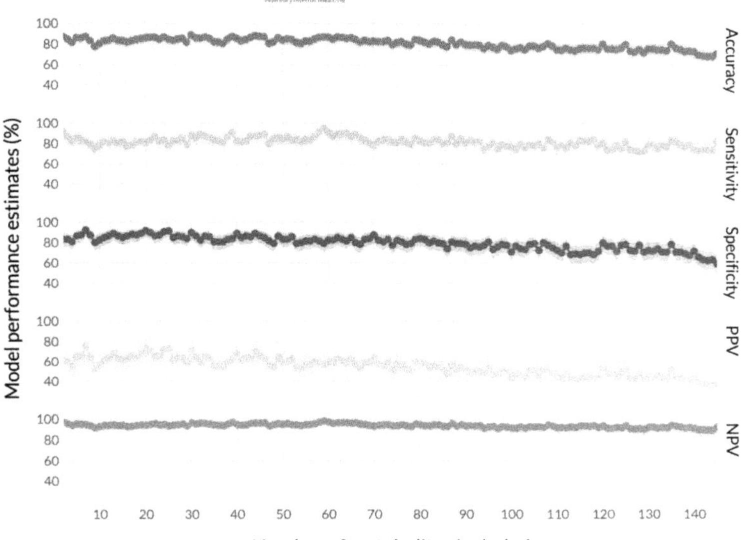

FIGURE 3 Model performance estimates on the baseline samples obtained by bootstrap cross-validation depending on the number of metabolites included. Positive Predictive Value (PPV) and Negative Predictive Value (NPV) were obtained using abovementioned formulas and the mean of previously reported prevalence of hyperinsulinemia.[28-30] The 95% confidence interval is shown as a shaded area behind each estimate. Overall, best model performance is reached with the top 7 and top 20 metabolites as determined by the baseline partial least-squares discriminant analysis (PLS-DA) model including all metabolites

An increase of Trp during the OGT previously has been reported in ponies,[17] whereas kynurenine was shown to increase in horses.[9] In our study, both molecules and their ratio (kynurenine : tryptophan) exhibited a positive concentration gradient, which might be attributable to enhanced indoleamine 2,3-dioxygenase (IDO) activity, considered to be induced by inflammatory processes and associated with metabolic syndrome in humans.[33] Thus, the OGT may elicit low-grade inflammation. Assuming the OGT models processes that occur naturally during grazing or nonstructural carbohydrate intake, this finding would support an inflammatory component in the pathogenesis of endocrinopathic laminitis, which could be responsible for chronic lamellar structural damage or priming metabolic pathomechanisms.

To our knowledge, an increase of DOPA (a precursor of dopamine) during the OGT has not been reported previously in any species. Parkinson's disease is associated with a loss of dopaminergic innervation in several brain areas, similar to the loss of dopaminergic inhibition in the *pars intermedia* of the pituitary gland of horses with PPID,[34] but also with glucose intolerance and diabetes.[35,36] A possible lack of inhibition of insulin secretion in β-cells of the pancreatic islets by DOPA and dopamine[37,38] could link the pathogenesis of PPID with ID.

4.2 | Differential response of insulin-dysregulated horses

Carnitine is necessary for the transportation of fatty acids into mitochondria for energy production via β-oxidation. Therefore, it has been hypothesized that obese individuals with higher plasma fatty acid concentrations use more carnitine.[39,40] In our study, a negative association between carnitine (C0) and the insulin response (AUC_{ins}; Figure 1B) was observed, possibly indicating similar differences in energy metabolism between hyper- and normo-insulinemic horses. Nevertheless, the benefits of carnitine supplementation were equivocal in this species.[41,42] Finally, if less carnitine is available for carnitine acetyltransferase, lower acetylcarnitine (C2) concentrations are to be expected (Figure 1B). The negative correlation between AUC_{ins} and acetylcarnitine observed in our study also emphasizes the importance of this metabolite in both PLS-DA models (Figure 2).

Arginine is another molecule available as a dietary supplement, and it is said to improve metabolic conditions such as obesity and Type-2 diabetes mellitus in rats, pigs, and humans.[43] Similar to its metabolites spermidine and putrescine, it was present in lower concentrations in horses with high insulin response (Figures 1B and 2). Arginine has been shown to increase oxidation of long-chain fatty acids and glucose,[43] but also is known for its strong vasodilatory effect, mediated by nitric oxide.[43,44] Lower arginine concentrations in horses with high insulin response therefore could be associated with some form of endothelial dysfunction, potentially involved in the pathophysiology of endocrinopathic laminitis.[45]

On the other hand, ADMA, the biologically active asymmetric stereoisomer of SDMA, which inhibits nitric oxide synthesis was slightly lower in horses with high insulin response (data not shown), and was given high importance in the 120 minutes PLS-DA model (Figure 2). Because SDMA and ADMA are derived from the catabolism of proteins containing methylated arginine, and not from methylation of free arginine,[46] the potential implications of this finding for the pathophysiology of ID remain obscure.

In our study, ID was assessed in a cut-off agnostic fashion using AUC_{ins} as an approximation of the total insulin response,[47,48] which encompasses basal HI and the response to glucose stimulation. The observed insulin responses at 120 minutes ranged from 20 to 240 μIU/mL. However, no horse was hyperinsulinemic at baseline[1] and insulin resistance was not assessed separately, whereas both factors could have impact on the metabolic phenotype. In addition, hypotheses have been made regarding the potential implications of some metabolites associated with a higher insulin response to glucose stimulation, but it remains unclear if these deviations are a cause or a consequence of ID.

4.3 | Classification performance and future perspectives

During the first PLS-DA approach, only 1 sample was excluded from each run of the model-training step and kept for model validation (leave-one-out-cross-validation). Therefore, compared to the second approach, where model metrics were obtained by bootstrap cross-validation, better model performance is achievable at the cost of a higher risk for overfitting.

Several metabolites not identified by the linear model approach had notable variable importance in projection (eg, SDMA, ADMA, Ala; Figure 2). The reason for this observation might be that AUC_{ins} was used as a continuous variable in the linear model, whereas it was dichotomized in the PLS-DA approach. Therefore, linear correlations might be masked whereas nonlinear relationships could be uncovered. Additionally, during PLS-DA, all metabolites were considered simultaneously, allowing detection of metabolites of predictive value in the scope of statistical interactions.

Because of the complexity and costs of metabolomics analysis, it does not appear feasible to use large metabolite panels for diagnostic purposes in animals. Therefore, we investigated the discriminatory potential of the panel while gradually decreasing the number of metabolites used, in order of descending variable importance from the initial baseline model. Our objective was to determine if similar accuracy was achievable using fewer metabolites, which could be brought to a different diagnostic platform, such as a multiplex point-of-care device. The results presented in Figure 3 are considered a proof-of-concept. The decrease in the number of metabolites appears beneficial to model performance. This finding possibly could be a result of the high dimensionality of the data (many more metabolites than samples), for which PLS-DA is more sensitive than other classification algorithms. However, because sample size was small and the interpretation limited to a proof-of-concept, it was considered best not to introduce additional statistical methods. Best model performance was reached at 7 and 20 metabolites, which, depending on the detection technique, can be considered a feasible number of analytes to include into a point-of-care device.[49]

In our study, the effect of artificial HI was investigated in a hypothesis-driven metabolomics approach. It remains to be confirmed if naturally occurring HI has similar metabolic impact. Several metabolites involved in inflammatory processes and vascular dysfunction, potentially involved in the pathogenesis of ID or laminitis, were identified. However, because laminitis was not induced during the study, additional experiments on larger cohorts are warranted.

5 | CONCLUSION

In our study, the response of horses to OGT was described on the metabolomic level. Results from previous experiments in horses were confirmed, but several new potential biomarkers for HI also were identified. Metabolites linked to β-oxidation (eg, acetylcarnitine, carnitine) were strongly associated with total insulin response. In addition, signs of a low-grade inflammatory response to the OGT (increased kynurenine : tryptophan) and potential vascular impairment associated with ID (decreased Arg and spermidine concentrations) were found. Oral supplementation of carnitine and Arg already have been used successfully against metabolic disorders in several species and could be investigated as potential therapeutic targets. Although confirmatory studies still are required, our results may aid in development of a point-of-care device to identify hyperinsulinemic horses using a single unstimulated blood sample.

ACKNOWLEDGMENTS

No funding was received for this study. The authors thank Professor Wolfgang Leibold for his support and providing the horses, and Dr Björn Steinbjörnsson for his help during the experiments and dedicated care to the horses.

CONFLICT OF INTEREST DECLARATION

Authors declare no conflict of interest.

OFF-LABEL ANTIMICROBIAL DECLARATION

Authors declare no off-label use of antimicrobials.

INSTITUTIONAL ANIMAL CARE AND USE COMMITTEE (IACUC) OR OTHER APPROVAL DECLARATION

The State Office for Consumer Protection and Food Safety (LAVES) approved the study in accordance with the German Animal Welfare Law (file number: 33.19-42 502-05-17A099).

HUMAN ETHICS APPROVAL DECLARATION

Authors declare human ethics approval was not needed for this study.

ORCID

Julien Delarocque https://orcid.org/0000-0002-4598-3499
Tobias Warnken https://orcid.org/0000-0002-0741-4674

REFERENCES

1. Frank N, Geor RJ, Bailey SR, Durham AE, Johnson PJ, American College of Veterinary Internal Medicine. Equine metabolic syndrome. *J Vet Intern Med*. 2010;24(3):467-475.
2. Frank N, Tadros EM. Insulin dysregulation. *Equine Vet J*. 2014;46(1):103-112.
3. Durham AE, Frank N, McGowan CM, et al. ECEIM consensus statement on equine metabolic syndrome. *J Vet Intern Med*. 2019;33(2):335-349.
4. Asplin KE, Sillence MN, Pollitt CC, McGowan CM. Induction of laminitis by prolonged hyperinsulinaemia in clinically normal ponies. *Vet J*. 2007;174(3):530-535.
5. de Laat MA, McGowan CM, Sillence MN, Pollitt CC. Equine laminitis: induced by 48 h hyperinsulinaemia in Standardbred horses. *Equine Vet J*. 2010;42(2):129-135.
6. Meier AD, de Laat MA, Reiche DB, et al. The oral glucose test predicts laminitis risk in ponies fed a diet high in nonstructural carbohydrates. *Domest Anim Endocrinol*. 2018;63(November):1-9.
7. Waller APP, Huettner L, Kohler K, Lacombe VAA. Novel link between inflammation and impaired glucose transport during equine insulin resistance. *Vet Immunol Immunopathol*. 2012;149(3-4):208-215.
8. Treiber K, Carter R, Gay L, Williams C, Geor R. Inflammatory and redox status of ponies with a history of pasture-associated laminitis. *Vet Immunol Immunopathol*. 2009;129(3-4):216-220.
9. Kenéz À, Warnken T, Feige K, Huber K. Lower plasma trans-4-hydroxyproline and methionine sulfoxide levels are associated with insulin dysregulation in horses. *BMC Vet Res*. 2018;14:146.
10. Bertin FR, de Laat MA. The diagnosis of equine insulin dysregulation. *Equine Vet J*. 2017;49(5):570-576.
11. Fitzgerald DM, Walsh DM, Sillence MN, Pollitt CC, de Laat MA. Insulin and incretin responses to grazing in insulin-dysregulated and healthy ponies. *J Vet Intern Med*. 2018;33(1):225-232.
12. Suagee JK, Corl BA, Crisman MV, Hulver MW, McCutcheon LJ, Geor RJ. Effects of acute hyperinsulinemia on inflammatory proteins in horses. *Vet Immunol Immunopathol*. 2011;142(3-4):141-146.
13. Banse HE, Frank N, Kwong GPS, McFarlane D. Relationship of oxidative stress in skeletal muscle with obesity and obesity-associated hyperinsulinemia in horses. *Can J Vet Res*. 2015;79(4):329-338.
14. Vick MM, Adams AA, Murphy BA, et al. Relationships among inflammatory cytokines, obesity, and insulin sensitivity in the horse. *J Anim Sci*. 2007;85(5):1144-1155.
15. Holbrook TC, Tipton T, McFarlane D. Neutrophil and cytokine dysregulation in hyperinsulinemic obese horses. *Vet Immunol Immunopathol*. 2012;145(1-2):283-289.
16. Kenéz À, Dänicke S, Rolle-Kampczyk U, von Bergen M, Huber K. A metabolomics approach to characterize phenotypes of metabolic transition from late pregnancy to early lactation in dairy cows. *Metabolomics*. 2016;12(11):1-11.
17. Jacob SI, Murray KJ, Rendahl AK, Geor RJ, Schultz NE, McCue ME. Metabolic perturbations in Welsh Ponies with insulin dysregulation, obesity, and laminitis. *J Vet Intern Med*. 2018;32(3):1215-1233.
18. Frank N, Andrews F, Durham A, et al. Recommendations for the diagnosis and treatment of pituitary pars intermedia dysfunction (PPID). 2015.
19. Öberg J, Bröjer J, Wattle O, Lilliehöök I. Evaluation of an equine-optimized enzyme-linked immunosorbent assay for serum insulin measurement and stability study of equine serum insulin. *Comp Clin Path*. 2011;21(6):1291-1300.
20. Pallares-Méndez R, Aguilar-Salinas CA, Cruz-Bautista I, Del Bosque-Plata L. Metabolomics in diabetes, a review. *Ann Med*. 2016;48(1-2):89-102.
21. Haucke V, Di Paolo G. Lipids and lipid modifications in the regulation of membrane traffic. *Curr Opin Cell Biol*. 2007;19(4):426-435.
22. Petersen MC, Shulman GI. Mechanisms of insulin action and insulin resistance. *Physiol Rev*. 2018;98(4):2133-2223.
23. Klein MS, Buttchereit N, Miemczyk SP, et al. NMR metabolomic analysis of dairy cows reveals milk glycerophosphocholine to phosphocholine ratio as prognostic biomarker for risk of ketosis. *J Proteome Res*. 2012;11(2):1373-1381.
24. Ding M, Rexrode KM. A review of lipidomics of cardiovascular disease highlights the importance of isolating lipoproteins. *Metabolites*. 2020;10(4):1-13.
25. Bolstad BM, Irizarry R, Astrand M, Speed TP. A comparison of normalization methods for high density oligonucleotide array data based on variance and bias. *Bioinformatics*. 2003;19(2):185-193.
26. Benjamini Y, Hochberg Y. Controlling the false discovery rate: a practical and powerful approach to multiple testing. *J R Stat Soc Ser B*. 1995;57:289-300.
27. Sanchez G. DiscriMiner: Tools of the Trade for Discriminant Analysis. 2013.
28. Muno JD. *Prevalence, Risk Factors and Seasonality of Plasma Insulin Concentrations in Normal Horses in Central Ohio*. Columbus, Ohio: The Ohio State University; 2009.
29. Pleasant RS, Suagee JK, Thatcher CD, Elvinger F, Geor RJ. Adiposity, plasma insulin, leptin, lipids, and oxidative stress in mature light breed horses. *J Vet Intern Med*. 2013;27(3):576-582.
30. Morgan RA, McGowan TW, Mcgowan CM. Prevalence and risk factors for hyperinsulinaemia in ponies in Queensland, Australia. *Aust Vet J*. 2014;92(4):101-106.
31. Ho JE, Larson MG, Vasan RS, et al. Metabolite profiles during oral glucose challenge. *Diabetes*. 2013;62(8):2689-2698.
32. Shaham O, Wei R, Wang TJ, et al. Metabolic profiling of the human response to a glucose challenge reveals distinct axes of insulin sensitivity. *Mol Syst Biol*. 2008;4(214):1-9.
33. Mangge H, Summers KL, Meinitzer A, et al. Obesity-related dysregulation of the Tryptophan-Kynurenine metabolism: role of age and parameters of the metabolic syndrome. *Obesity*. 2014;22(1):195-201.
34. Millington WR, Dybdal NO, Dawson R, Manzini C, Mueller GP. Equine Cushing's disease: differential regulation of β-endorphin processing in tumors of the intermediate pituitary. *Endocrinology*. 1988;123(3):1598-1604.
35. Lipman IJ, Boykin ME, Flora RE. Glucose intolerance in Parkinson's disease. *J Chronic Dis*. 1974;27:573-579.
36. Santiago JA, Potashkin JA. Shared dysregulated pathways lead to Parkinson's disease and diabetes. *Trends Mol Med*. 2013;19(3):176-186.
37. Lundquist I, Panagiotidis G, Stenstrom A. Effect of L-DOPA administration on islet monoamine oxidase activity and glucose-induced insulin release in the mouse. *Pancreas*. 1991;6(5):522-527.
38. Boyd AE, Lebovitz HE, Feldman JM. Endocrine function and glucose metabolism in patients with Parkinson's disease and their alteration by L-dopa. *J Clin Endocrinol Metab*. 1971;33(5):829-837.
39. Xie B, Waters MJ, Schirra HJ. Investigating potential mechanisms of obesity by metabolomics. *J Biomed Biotechnol*. 2012;2012:1-10.
40. Seiler SE, Martin OJ, Noland RC, et al. Obesity and lipid stress inhibit carnitine acetyltransferase activity. *J Lipid Res*. 2014;55(4):635-644.
41. Van Weyenberg S, Buyse J, Janssens GPJ. Increased plasma leptin through l-carnitine supplementation is associated with an enhanced glucose tolerance in healthy ponies. *J Anim Physiol Anim Nutr*. 2009;93(2):203-208.
42. Morgan R, Keen J, McGowan C. Equine metabolic syndrome. *Vet Rec*. 2015;177(7):173-179.

43. McKnight JR, Satterfield MC, Jobgen WS, et al. Beneficial effects of L-arginine on reducing obesity: potential mechanisms and important implications for human health. *Amino Acids*. 2010;39(2):349-357.
44. Bode-Böger SM. Effect of L-arginine supplementation on NO production in man. *Eur J Clin Pharmacol*. 2006;62(Suppl. 13):91-99.
45. Morgan RA, Keen JA, Walker BR, Hadoke PWF. Vascular dysfunction in horses with endocrinopathic laminitis. *PLoS One*. 2016;11(9):1-14.
46. Cooke JP. Does ADMA cause endothelial dysfunction? *Arterioscler Thromb Vasc Biol*. 2000;20(9):2032-2037.
47. Dühlmeier R, Deegen E, Fuhrmann H, et al. Glucose-dependent insulinotropic polypeptide (GIP) and the enteroinsular axis in equines (*Equus caballus*). *Comp Biochem Physiol A Mol Integr Physiol*. 2001;129 (2-3):563-575.
48. Lerner RL, Porte D. Relationships between intravenous glucose loads, insulin responses and glucose disappearance rate. *J Clin Endocrinol Metab*. 1971;33(3):409-417.
49. Dincer C, Bruch R, Kling A, Dittrich PS, Urban GA. Multiplexed point-of-care testing – xPOCT. *Trends Biotechnol*. 2017;35(8):728-742.
50. Ritchie Matthew E., Phipson Belinda, Wu Di, Hu Yifang, Law Charity W., Shi Wei, Smyth Gordon K.. limma powers differential expression analyses for RNA-sequencing and microarray studies. *Nucleic Acids Research*. 2015;43 (7):e47–e47. http://dx.doi.org/10.1093/nar/gkv007.

SUPPORTING INFORMATION

Additional supporting information may be found online in the Supporting Information section at the end of this article.

How to cite this article: Delarocque J, Frers F, Feige K, Huber K, Jung K, Warnken T. Metabolic changes induced by oral glucose tests in horses and their diagnostic use. *J Vet Intern Med*. 2020;1–9. https://doi.org/10.1111/jvim.15992

Supporting information

Appendix S1 Detailed description of the methods used for statistical analysis.

Statistical analysis

Statistical analysis was performed with R 3.6.0 [1].

The metabolomics dataset was prepared by removing metabolites with more than 50% of values below the limit of detection (LOD). Remaining values below LOD were set to LOD/2. After aligning the measurement batches by QC-RLSC [2], metabolites with CV over 20% were removed. After log_2-transformation, batch and trial effect were removed using the 'removeBacthEffect' function from the limma package [3]. Then, the data were scaled (auto-scaling), quantile normalized [4] and checked for outliers using the 'bagplot' method [5]. The explanatory variables Age and Area Under the Curve of Insulin (AUC_{ins} – approximating the total insulin response to OGT) were log_2-transformed.

Analysis of differential concentration was conducted with the limma package [3] with the aim of identifying associations between each metabolite and factors like time of the OGT or level of insulin dysregulation (AUC_{ins}). A linear model including time of the OGT (0, 120 or 180 min) and AUC_{ins} as continuous predictors, adjusted for age and sex, was defined. To account for repeated measures, 'horse' was added as blocking factor and the intra-individual correlation taken into account by the model. Resulting p-values were adjusted to control a False Discovery Rate (FDR) of 5 % using the Benjamini-Hochberg procedure [6].

For predictive modelling, partial least squares discriminant analysis (PLS-DA) [7] was performed using the DiscriMiner package [8]. To determine if a set of some metabolites included in the assay could be used to differentiate horses with high and low insulin quantities, the AUC_{ins} was partitioned in two groups of same size ('HIGH' and 'LOW'). A PLS-DA with leave-one-out-cross-validation (LOOCV) was run separately on the baseline and 120 min samples separately with all metabolites included to determine the variable importance of each metabolite.

In a second approach, the number of metabolites included in the baseline classifier model was varied as hyper-parameter during a bootstrap cross-validation. The order of removal of metabolites was the increasing order of metabolite importance as determined in the initial baseline model (see above). Twenty random subsets of 15 samples per group where taken each time as training data. Using the remaining samples as test data, different estimators of model performance (sensitivity, specificity, accuracy, Positive Predictive Value [PPV] and Negative Predictive Value [NPV]) were calculated. Ninety-five percent confidence intervals of these estimators where determined using the Clopper and Pearson method on the sums of the confusion matrices obtained by validation in each resampling. As the prevalence of hyperinsulinemia in the study population might not reflect the prevalence in the general population, the positive and negative predictive value estimated by the confusion matrices could be biased. Therefore PPV and NPV were estimated using **Formulas 1** and **2** respectively with prevalence set at the mean value of 22.5 % from the prevalence reported by three distinct studies [9–11]. The methodological differences between these studies were not accounted for.

$$PPV = \frac{Sensitivity \times Prevalence}{Sensitivity \times Prevalence + (1 - Specificity) \times (1 - Prevalence)} \quad (1)$$

$$NPV = \frac{Specificity \times (1 - Prevalence)}{(1 - Sensitivity) \times Prevalence + Specificity \times (1 - Prevalence)} \quad (2)$$

References

[1] R Core Team. R: A Language and Environment for Statistical Computing 2020.

[2] Dunn WB, Broadhurst D, Begley P, Zelena E, Francis-Mcintyre S, Anderson N, et al. Procedures for large-scale metabolic profiling of serum and plasma using gas chromatography and liquid chromatography coupled to mass spectrometry. Nat Protoc 2011;6:1060–83.

[3] Ritchie ME, Phipson B, Wu D, Hu Y, Law CW, Shi W, et al. limma powers differential expression analyses for RNA-sequencing and microarray studies. Nucleic Acids Res 2015;43:e47–e47.

[4] Bolstad BM, Irizarry R., Astrand M, Speed TP. A comparison of normalization methods for high density oligonucleotide array data based on variance and bias. Bioinformatics 2003;19:185–93.

[5] Kruppa J, Jung K. Automated multigroup outlier identification in molecular high-throughput data using bagplots and gemplots. BMC Bioinformatics 2017;18:1–10.

[6] Benjamini Y, Hochberg Y. Controlling the False Discovery Rate: A Practical and Powerful Approach to Multiple Testing. J R Stat Soc Ser B 1995;57:289–300.

[7] Barker M, Rayens W. Partial least squares for discrimination. J Chemom 2003;17:166–73.

[8] Sanchez G. DiscriMiner: Tools of the Trade for Discriminant Analysis 2013.

[9] Muno JD. Prevalence, risk factors and seasonality of plasma insulin concentrations in normal horses in central Ohio. The Ohio State University, 2009.

[10] Pleasant RSS, Suagee JKK, Thatcher CDD, Elvinger F, Geor RJJ. Adiposity, plasma insulin, leptin, lipids, and oxidative stress in mature light breed horses. J Vet Intern Med 2013;27:576–82.

[11] Morgan RA, McGowan TW, Mcgowan CM. Prevalence and risk factors for hyperinsulinaemia in ponies in Queensland, Australia. Aust Vet J 2014;92:101–6.

Table S1 Table listing the VIP scores of each metabolite in the full baseline PLS-DA model. In the reduced PLS-DA models, the metabolites were removed by order of increasing VIP score (e.g., the reduced model with two metabolites included only C2 and SDMA as predictors).

Metabolite	VIP Score	Rank	Metabolite	VIP Score	Rank
C2	2,8757603	1	PC aa C38:0	0,812634407	74
SDMA	2,300430375	2	lysoPC a C20:4	0,795023423	75
acylcarnitines	2,266748393	3	SM (OH) C22:1	0,771084337	76
PC aa C40:4	2,196393733	4	SM C26:1	0,755159734	77
Putrescine	2,001274243	5	Thr	0,750395208	78
ADMA	1,931177915	6	aminoacids	0,738978787	79
PC aa C40:3	1,764873754	7	PC ae C38:5	0,736620543	80
C14:1	1,750783052	8	C5	0,729537961	81
Ala	1,71755374	9	PC ae C36:3	0,716363379	82
PC aa C40:6	1,669523913	10	PC aa C36:6	0,714773447	83
PC aa C40:2	1,645988592	11	PC ae C40:2	0,703444059	84
PC aa C28:1	1,587090741	12	lysoPC a C18:2	0,702716091	85
t4-OH-Pro	1,582084455	13	Phe	0,701361328	86
C16	1,558400511	14	biogenic amines	0,697540317	87
Cit	1,519437882	15	lysoPC a C16:0	0,662379113	88
c4-OH-Pro	1,493385166	16	Histamine	0,654804501	89
Creatinine	1,482084665	17	PC aa C38:6	0,632058608	90
PC ae C40:6	1,461073066	18	SM (OH) C22:2	0,629637299	91
PC ae C34:1	1,449120211	19	PC ae C32:2	0,600242367	92
PC aa C40:5	1,432990502	20	Tyr	0,579155435	93
lysoPC a C24:0	1,420661028	21	SM C26:0	0,577731746	94
PC aa C38:4	1,388708862	22	His	0,574480638	95
Dopamine	1,383092264	23	KynTrp	0,57111279	96
Gln	1,381517846	24	PC aa C32:3	0,570156063	97
PC ae C38:4	1,32304449	25	PC ae C40:4	0,569484856	98
Met	1,30616121	26	SM C18:0	0,562702246	99
C4	1,288050243	27	PC ae C36:0	0,558379236	100
PC ae C38:2	1,284034448	28	PC aa C32:0	0,554793624	101
Spermidine	1,283248985	29	SM C16:1	0,553985231	102
lysoPC a C28:1	1,229721618	30	PC ae C36:5	0,550235377	103
PC ae C42:4	1,201620014	31	PC ae C32:1	0,547613564	104
PC ae C36:1	1,188673265	32	H1	0,542812236	105
Asn	1,181332591	33	Taurine	0,49536266	106
PC aa C34:2	1,180969277	34	PC ae C34:0	0,491907934	107
Asp	1,160434305	35	lysoPC a C18:0	0,491359344	108
Pro	1,149668192	36	PC aa C34:4	0,491205242	109
PC ae C38:1	1,13921199	37	Val	0,485094718	110
DOPA	1,127939469	38	Serotonin	0,480736956	111
PC aa C32:2	1,110150128	39	PC aa C30:0	0,467875158	112
PC aa C30:2	1,109932947	40	C0	0,464064142	113

PC aa C38:5	1,08202271	41
PC ae C40:5	1,077120195	42
PC ae C38:0	1,068386994	43
PEA	1,046835035	44
PC aa C42:1	1,036074828	45
PC aa C32:1	1,034401105	46
glycerophospholipids	1,018603352	47
PC aa C34:1	1,006786838	48
SM C20:2	0,987279041	49
PC aa C36:5	0,974148664	50
SM (OH) C16:1	0,964979125	51
Trp	0,963326003	52
PC aa C34:3	0,960232248	53
alpha-AAA	0,955167679	54
PC ae C38:6	0,950984036	55
PC aa C42:6	0,945001282	56
lysoPC a C28:0	0,94011556	57
PC ae C42:2	0,910095651	58
SM C18:1	0,909580692	59
Arg	0,891853649	60
Ser	0,891623715	61
Gly	0,887327407	62
PC ae C42:3	0,864274517	63
PC aa C42:5	0,86399434	64
PC aa C36:1	0,863155993	65
Glu	0,855537953	66
PC ae C40:1	0,85048145	67
lysoPC a C16:1	0,8399183	68
PC aa C38:3	0,827263983	69
PC ae C40:3	0,824933077	70
PC ae C38:3	0,821174151	71
Met-SO	0,813681257	72
PC aa C36:3	0,812777866	73

PC aa C42:4	0,444756441	114
Nitro-Tyr	0,442108039	115
PC ae C30:2	0,399320491	116
Spermine	0,392773106	117
PC ae C36:2	0,389847577	118
sphingolipids	0,367479179	119
Kynurenine	0,367004304	120
lysoPC a C17:0	0,353673273	121
PC ae C34:3	0,350329292	122
SM C24:0	0,346305275	123
Ile	0,345239632	124
PC aa C40:1	0,34307653	125
Orn	0,34228588	126
PC aa C36:2	0,340099792	127
Sarcosine	0,331144136	128
SM C22:3	0,330551196	129
PC ae C44:3	0,326723441	130
Leu	0,313732899	131
Lys	0,307392819	132
SM (OH) C14:1	0,307232349	133
PC aa C38:1	0,267493944	134
SM C16:0	0,258816784	135
lysoPC a C18:1	0,251397915	136
SM C24:1	0,243509156	137
C3	0,239759386	138
PC aa C36:4	0,231461116	139
Carnosine	0,199626707	140
SM (OH) C24:1	0,176457497	141
PC ae C34:2	0,169319516	142
PC ae C36:4	0,158732258	143
PC ae C44:6	0,147449844	144
PC ae C30:0	0,05675758	145

3. Manuscript 2

Weight loss is linearly associated with a reduction of the insulin response to an oral glucose test in Icelandic horses

Julien Delarocque[1]*, Florian Frers[1], Korinna Huber[2], Karsten Feige[1], Tobias Warnken[1]

[1] Clinic for Horses, University of Veterinary Medicine Hannover, Foundation, Hannover, Germany.

[2] Institute of Animal Science, Faculty of Agricultural Sciences, University of Hohenheim, Stuttgart, Germany.

* Corresponding author

State of publication:

Published in BMC Veterinary Research (2020) 16:151
DOI: 10.1186/s12917-020-02356-w

Contributions to the manuscript:

T. Warnken and K. Feige designed the experiments. J. Delarocque and F. Frers performed the experiments. J. Delarocque measured the insulin concentrations, analysed the data, prepared the figures and wrote the manuscript. J. Delarocque, F. Frers, K. Huber, K. Feige and T. Warnken contributed to the interpretation of the results and reviewed drafts of the manuscript. All authors read and accepted the final manuscript.

Delarocque *et al. BMC Veterinary Research* (2020) 16:151
https://doi.org/10.1186/s12917-020-02356-w

BMC Veterinary Research

RESEARCH ARTICLE

Open Access

Weight loss is linearly associated with a reduction of the insulin response to an oral glucose test in Icelandic horses

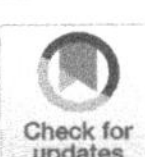

Julien Delarocque[1*], Florian Frers[1], Korinna Huber[2], Karsten Feige[1] and Tobias Warnken[1]

Abstract

Background: Insulin dysregulation (ID) goes along with lasting or transient hyperinsulinemia able to trigger equine laminitis, a painful and crippling foot condition. Promoting weight loss through dietary changes and physical activity is currently the main option to prevent this disease. This study aimed at describing the relationship between weight variations and the level of ID as determined by oral glucose tests (OGT). Therefore, the insulin response of 19 Icelandic horses to repeated OGTs was retrospectively analysed considering the variations in their body weight.

Results: There was a strong linear relationship between variations in body weight and variations in the total insulin response to OGT as approximated by the area under the curve of insulin ($p < 0.001$). As indicated by a weighted least squares model, the insulin response decreased by 22% for 5% weight loss on average. However some horses did not respond to weight loss with a reduction of their insulin response to OGT. Additionally, a high correlation between 120 min serum insulin concentration and total insulin response was observed ($r = 0.96$, $p < 0.001$).

Conclusions: The results corroborate that weight loss is effective against ID and allow for a better quantification of the expected improvement of the insulin response after weight loss. However, it is unclear why some horses did not respond as expected. The high correlation between the 120 min insulin concentration and total insulin response suggests that insulin status can be accurately determined and monitored with only few samples in a practical setting.

Keywords: Insulin dysregulation, Equine metabolic syndrome, Weight loss, Obesity, Oral glucose test, Laminitis, Horse

Background

Since obesity was identified as a risk factor for laminitis [1, 2], the metabolic health of obese horses has been studied intensively. Eventually, the Equine Metabolic Syndrome (EMS) was defined as a collection of risk factors for this disease, among which insulin dysregulation (ID) plays a major role [3–5]. The term ID encompasses insulin resistance (IR), exaggerated insulin response to oral carbohydrates and fasting hyperinsulinemia (HI) and therefore results in either permanent or transient HI. As HI was shown to induce laminitis [6, 7], it was sought to increase insulin sensitivity (SI) in horses affected by EMS through various weight loss programs [8]. These more or less complex programs relied on increased physical activity [9, 10], restricted energy intake [11–15] or both [15–17]. While combined programs were effective, SI did not necessarily improve when either activity or dietary changes were absent [9, 10, 15]. However, comparing these studies is challenging, because of dissimilar methodologies and a vast number of involved variables (e.g. breed, age, energy source, exact energy intake and expense, etc.). Moreover, it was

* Correspondence: julien.delarocque@tiho-hannover.de
[1]Clinic for Horses, University of Veterinary Medicine Hannover, Foundation, Bünteweg 9, 30559 Hanover, Germany
Full list of author information is available at the end of the article

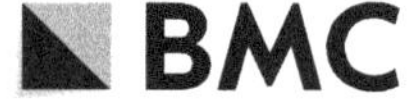

suggested that obesity is not in itself responsible for a reduced SI in horses [18], which is consistent with the description of a lean EMS phenotype [5, 19] and supports the existence of contributing factors to EMS distinct from IR and obesity.

As HI also occurs in insulin sensitive horses [19, 20], the assessment of SI – a measure associated with IR – is probably insufficient to evaluate the effects of weight loss on ID. While the term ID had not been introduced at that time, the effect of weight loss on the area under the curve of insulin over time (AUC_{ins}) during an oral glucose test (OGT) has already been investigated by Van Weyenberg et al. in 2008 [11]. The AUC_{ins}, which can be seen as an approximation of the total quantity of insulin secreted during a period of time [21, 22], is a good descriptor of the level of HI induced by a carbohydrate challenge. Further was the use of an oral testing protocol judicious, since these are sensitive to all aspects of ID, contrary to intravenous tests [5].

Five Oral Glucose Tests (OGT) were conducted in 19 Icelandic horses over 1 year during a longitudinal study. As substantial variations in body weight were noticed, it was retrospectively decided to describe the relationship between weight variations and insulin response within each horse to investigate the effect of weight loss on ID.

Results

Weight and AUC_{ins} variations

All horses lost weight over the year ($p < 0.001$). However, the body weight did not monotonically decrease in all individuals. The median maximal weight difference observed within one horse was 12% (45 kg) on the large pasture and 11% (41 kg) on the small pasture. No overall pasture differences were found ($p > 0.9$). The pasture-time interaction ($p = 0.004$) resulted in a significant difference at only one OGT (Fig. 1).

Variations within time were also present for $rAUC_{ins}$ ($p = 0.004$) but no effect of pasture was observed either ($p > 0.9$). The pasture-time interaction ($p = 0.03$) was associated with a significant difference at a single OGT ($p = 0.01$) (Fig. 1).

Relationship between relative weight and relative area under the curve of insulin over time

In a first model with no distinction of pastures, the relative insulin response, as approximated by $rAUC_{ins}$, was significantly predicted by rWeight ($\beta = 4.4$, SE = 0.6, AIC = 91.9, Number of observations = 95, $p < 0.001$). Overall, 5% weight loss were associated with a reduction of the insulin response of 22%. The addition of pasture to the model improved model fit ($X^2(2) = 16$, $p < 0.001$). The effect of rWeight increased ($\beta = 5.3$, SE = 0.6, AIC = 79.8, Number of observations = 95, $p < 0.001$) but was inversed for the small pasture ($\beta = -6.4$, SE = 1.4, $p < 0.001$). The effect of pasture was significant as well ($\beta = 6.4$, SE = 1.4, $p < 0.001$). As a result, 5% weight loss were associated with a reduction of the insulin response of 26% for horses on the large pasture and an increase of the insulin response of 5% on the small one (Fig. 2). The regression slopes are compared with individual trends in Fig. 3.

Correlation between the area under the curve of insulin over time with the serum insulin concentration at 120 min

The AUC_{ins} and $[Insulin]_{120}$ expressed a strong linear correlation ($r = 0.96$) (Fig. 4).

Discussion

The aim of this study was to describe the relationship between weight variations and the insulin response to a glucose challenge. Over a period of nearly 1 year, 19 horses were weighed and subjected to OGTs at regular intervals. Important weight variations – mostly weight loss – were observed. These variations are attributable to unmonitored changes in feed quality and voluntary physical activity. The relative weight significantly predicted the insulin response with 5% weight loss being associated with a reduction of the insulin response of 22%.

When comparing the regression slopes of the relative body weight against the relative insulin response to the trend within individuals (Fig. 3), four horses showing no reduction of the insulin response despite weight loss can easily be identified. These horses came from the smaller pasture, together with horse 3, which was the only stallion. As a conclusion, the causes for the variations in the response to weight loss took place either on the individual level or on pasture level but were compensated by individual factors (like sex) in one horse. By fitting a distinct slope for each pasture, the effect of weight loss became more apparent for horses from the larger pasture, displaying a reduction of the insulin response of 26% for 5% weight loss (Fig. 2).

Possible causes for the lack of response in some individuals

Neither the evolution of the relative body weight nor of the relative insulin response follow a radically different trend over time between pastures (Fig. 1). When looking at absolute values (data not shown), no statistically significant differences were found between pastures within OGTs. Therefore, the lack of response in most individuals of the smaller pasture appears not to be related to a form of weight loss resistance [13] or a fundamentally higher level of insulin dysregulation, that would be refractory to weight loss. Nevertheless, changing proportions of metabolic active tissues depending on the level of physical activity (e.g. relatively more muscle and less

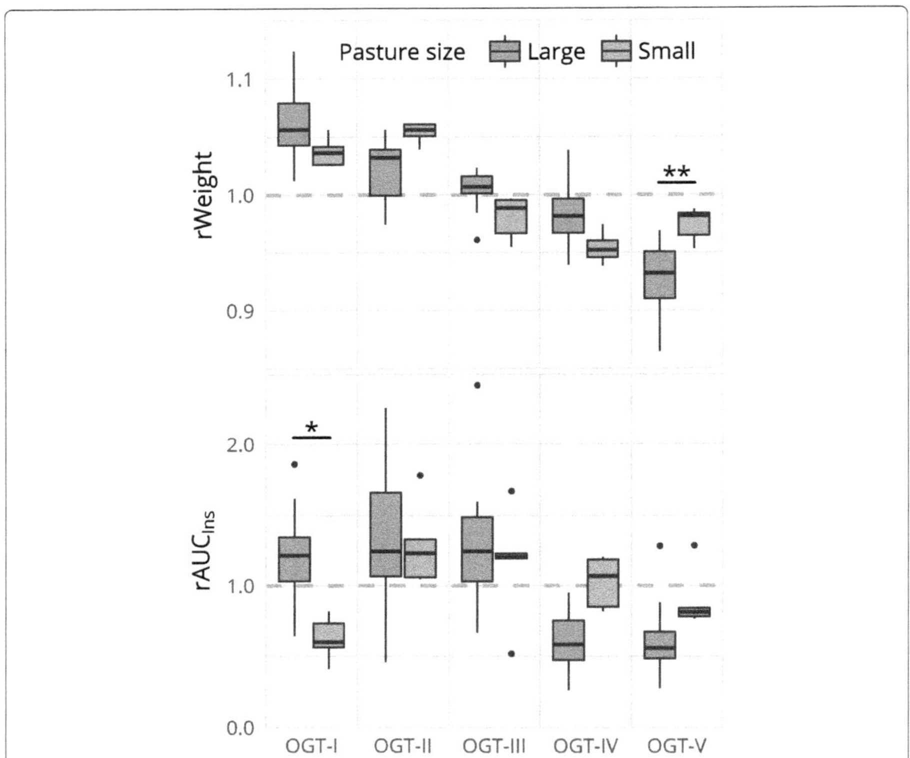

Fig. 1 Variation in time of the relative weight (rWeight) and relative area under the insulin curve ($rAUC_{Ins}$). The grey dotted line represents the mean weight resp. $rAUC_{Ins}$ over the year. The pairwise comparisons between groups for rWeight and $rAUC_{Ins}$ reveal that significant differences can only be found at one OGT in each case. However, no significant overall group differences were observed

white adipose tissue) could have an influence on the reduction of the insulin response without affecting body weight [23, 24].

Some differences exist in the age and sex distribution between groups. However, the younger group (small pasture) not responding to weight loss appears counterintuitive, since age seems to be positively associated with hyperinsulinemia [25] while sex does not [26]. Yet on the small pasture, the stallion responded to weight loss in contrast to the geldings (Fig. 3), so that there might be an effect of sex on the unknown factor confounded by pasture.

Even though differences in feeding are largely excluded (see Material and methods), there might have been dissimilarities regarding the preferably consumed feed (pasture grasses or hay) or an interaction between body condition and feed intake (both in quantity and quality) [27] that might in turn have affected ID or IR [25, 28–30].

Since there were more feeding places than horses on each pasture, an effect of herd hierarchy on available feed appears less likely. Nevertheless, hierarchy could have influenced energy expenditure [27]. As would have the slightly different density of horses on each pasture. Additionally, the layout of the pastures (Fig. 5) differs in such a way that the larger group could have undertaken more voluntary physical exercise than the small one by traveling from the pasture to the shelter several times over the day. The difference in exercising levels would

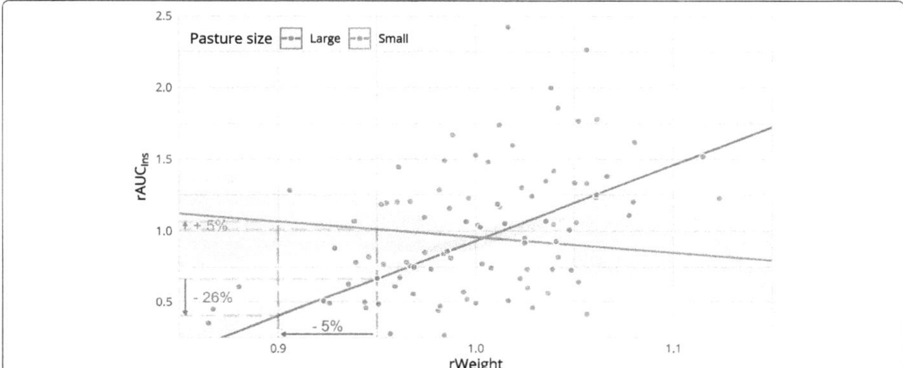

Fig. 2 Scatterplot representing the relationship between the relative weight (rWeight) and the relative AUC_{ins} ($rAUC_{ins}$). The regression lines with 95% CI from the weighted least squares model are presented in blue for the larger pasture and in red for the smaller one. On the large pasture a reduction of the relative weight of 5% led to a reduction of the $rAUC_{ins}$ of 26%, while in the other group the insulin response was rather stationary despite weight loss

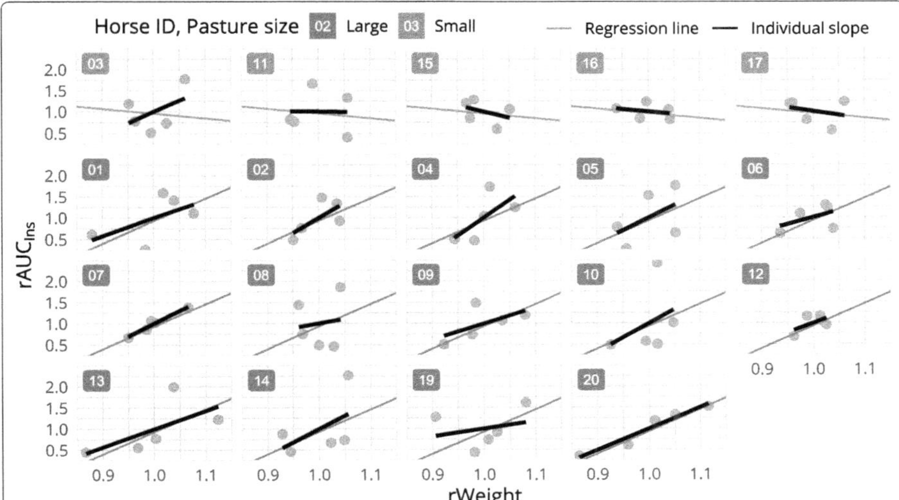

Fig. 3 Scatterplot of the relative weight (rWeight) and associated relative AUC_{ins} ($rAUC_{ins}$) for every horse. The coloured lines correspond to the regression lines of the full weighted least squares model presented in Fig. 2. The black line is the individual trend as determined by simple linear regression. On the small pasture the average evolution of the insulin response to weight loss is almost stationary, except for horse 3, whose response is rather similar to the one observed on the large pasture. Possible reasons for these differences by pastures are discussed in "Possible causes for the lack of response in some individuals"

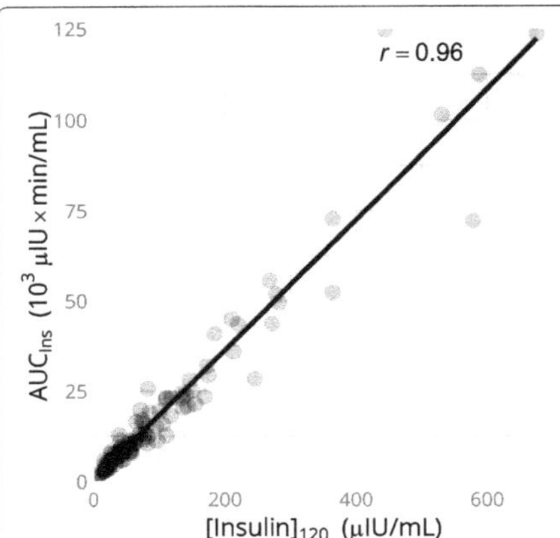

Fig. 4 Correlation between the AUC_{ins} and the serum insulin concentration at 120 min ($[Insulin]_{120}$). The correlation between both variables is very high ($r = 0.96$, $p < 0.001$), suggesting that the 120 min value can be used instead of the AUC_{ins} to assess the insulin response to glucose challenges without substantial loss of information

then be responsible for the differences in the response to weight loss. While this corroborates observations from the authors, these differences are not quantifiable due to the retrospective nature of the study. Previous studies have shown, that in the absence of physical activity, an increase of SI through weight loss cannot always be achieved [15]. However, a more stringent diet might help achieve satisfactory results without concurrent exercise [11]. Initial body weight and condition, genotype and the quality of provided forages [13, 31] might explain some differences between these studies. In human medicine, there is also discordant evidence regarding the relative importance of weight loss and exercise in improving SI [32–35].

Lastly, as insulin resistance was not assessed, it cannot be excluded that the horses of either of the groups were less sensitive to insulin, while dysregulated to a similar extent.

Practical relevance

Standardized testing protocols like the OGT do not induce laminitis. It is therefore difficult to quantify the reduction of insulinaemia required to confer a protection against endocrinopathic laminitis. It has been reported that the $[Insulin]_{120}$ measured during an OGT performed with 0.75 g/kg bwt glucose correlated well with the same measure during grazing, while slightly overestimating the insulin response [36]. The lower glucose dosage (0.5 g/kg bwt) used in this study possibly alleviates this bias, so that a reduction of the insulin response to grazing through weight loss and increased physical activity roughly similar to the reduction observed in the OGT with 0.5 g/kg bwt glucose can reasonably be expected.

In view of the high correlation between $[Insulin]_{120}$ and AUC_{ins} and the linear relationship between rWeight and $rAUC_{ins}$, monitoring the body weight after an initial 0.5 g/kg OGT with only two blood samples (basal and 120 min) could be sufficient to evaluate the evolution of ID. As the implementation of weight loss programs under field conditions might be difficult because of a lack of recognition of obesity [37], concerns regarding welfare under dietary restrictions [5], difficulties in implementing the measures in boarding stables and overall owner compliance [17], the simplified OGT can be repeated to ascertain the effectivity of the measures actually carried out.

Considerations on the study design and data analysis

Considering the AUC_{ins} an approximation of the level of HI corresponds better to our current understanding of the

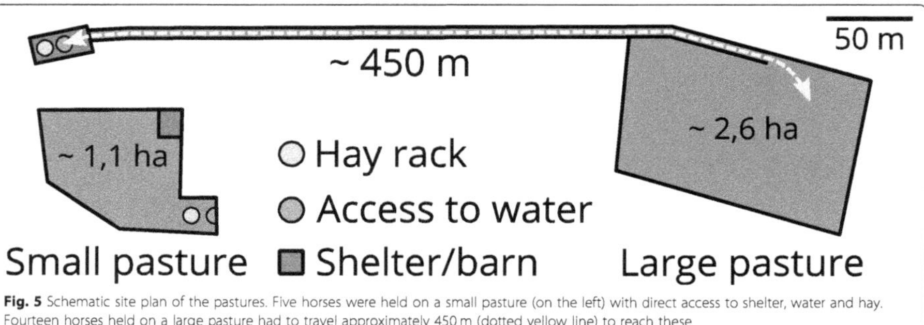

Fig. 5 Schematic site plan of the pastures. Five horses were held on a small pasture (on the left) with direct access to shelter, water and hay. Fourteen horses held on a large pasture had to travel approximately 450 m (dotted yellow line) to reach these

pathophysiology of ID than the oversimplistic categorisation of healthy and insulin-dysregulated individuals relying on a cut-off. Therefore, no target value to be reached can be given to set up weight loss programs. However safe levels can be determined in weight gain trials [38].

Further limitations are that a rather small and homogeneous population of horses was used and that no quantification of exercise nor diet changes could be performed due to the retrospective nature of the study. As individual variations in the response to weight reduction programs are high [13], it is however not necessarily detrimental to rely on the weight actually lost – which can be measured objectively – rather than estimating the energy expense induced by such programs to predict the reduction in the total insulin response. Lastly, both the magnitude of the correlation between the 120 min insulin concentration and total insulin response, and the nature and strength of the relationship between weight variations and insulin response might differ when other protocols for the OGT than the one described above are used.

Conclusion

To the authors' knowledge, this is the first study to demonstrate the linear relationship between the insulin response to a glucose challenge and the weight variations within individuals. These results corroborate the efficacy of weight loss against insulin dysregulation and are relevant for the prevention of laminitis and monitoring of insulin-dysregulated horses in a practical setting.

Methods

Horses

Nineteen university owned Icelandic horses of mixed metabolic status were enrolled in this project. For practical reasons five horses (1 stallion, 4 geldings; median age: 17 years, range: 9–17 years) were held as a small herd and fourteen horses (11 mares, 3 geldings; median age: 21 years, range: 14–29 years) were held as a large herd. Over the day, each group had access to neighbouring pastures similar in type and grass abundance (Fig. 5) and were fed hay from the same batches ad libitum. At the end of the experiment, the horses remained in their respective herds.

Weighing

The horses were weighed 9 to 16 days prior to each OGT with a mobile weighing scale (accuracy: 1%, resolution: 1 kg, precision: 2 kg).

Oral glucose tests

The OGTs were conducted on site five times at even intervals over a one-year period. The horses were fasted overnight for 8 h before the start of the experiments. In the morning, a jugular vein catheter was aseptically placed for blood collection. After a basal sample had been drawn, 0.5 g/kg bwt glucose were administered via nasogastric tube [39]. Further blood samples were collected 30, 60, 120, 180, and 240 min later. After collection, the samples were immediately transferred into VACUETTE® Serum Clot Activator Tubes.[1] They were left to clot at room temperature for 20–40 min and then kept at 4 °C. Within 6 h, all samples were centrifuged, aliquoted and stored at − 80 °C until further analysis.

Insulin measurements

Serum insulin concentrations were measured in duplicates at the end of the experimental phase using an equine-optimized ELISA (Mercodia Equine Insulin ELISA[2]; inter-assay CV 7.7%) previously validated for use in horses [40].

Statistical analysis

Statistical analysis was performed with R 3.6.1 [41] using the packages afex [42], nlme [43] and emmeans [44]. The area under the insulin curve over time (AUC_{ins}) was calculated using the trapezoidal method. The relative weight (rWeight) and the relative AUC_{ins} ($rAUC_{ins}$), both defined as the ratio of the weight or AUC_{ins} of the horse at one OGT to the mean weight or AUC_{ins} of this horse across all OGTs, were used for subsequent analysis to make the results comparable between horses.

A weighted least squares model with individual-level autocorrelation and OGT-level (number of trial) variance structure was fitted to the data with the maximum likelihood procedure using rWeight as single predictor of $rAUC_{ins}$. In a second model, the effect of 'Pasture' was added with a Pasture:rWeight interaction. Both models were compared by a likelihood ratio test. Normality of the residuals was ensured visually. Significance level was set at 0.05.

Repeated measures two-way ANOVA was used additionally to describe the evolution of rWeight and $rAUC_{ins}$ over time within and between groups independently. Post-hoc comparisons between groups within time were corrected for multiple comparisons using the Dunnett method.

The correlation between AUC_{ins} and serum insulin concentration at 120 min was assessed using the Pearson correlation coefficient.

[1]Greiner Bio-One International GmbH, Maybachstraße 2, D-72636 Frickenhausen, Germany

[2]Mercodia AB, Sylveniusgatan 8A, SE-754 50 Uppsala, Sweden

Abbreviations

AUC_{ins}: Area under the insulin curve over time; CV: Coefficient of variation; EMS: Equine Metabolic Syndrome; ID: Insulin dysregulation; IR: Insulin Resistance; OGT: Oral Glucose Test; $rAUC_{ins}$: Area under the insulin curve relatively to the mean area under the insulin curve of this horse; rWeight: Body weight relatively to the mean body weight of this horse.; SI: Insulin Sensitivity

Acknowledgements

The authors wish to thank Professor Wolfgang Leibold for his support and providing the horses, and Dr. Björn Steinbjörnsson for his help during the experiments and dedicated care to the horses.

Authors' contributions

TW and KF designed the experiments. JD and FF performed the experiments. JD measured the insulin concentrations, analysed the data, prepared the figures and wrote the manuscript. JD, FF, KH, KF and TW contributed to the interpretation of the results and reviewed drafts of the manuscript. All authors read and accepted the final manuscript.

Funding

No funding was received.

Availability of data and materials

The dataset analysed during the current study is available from the corresponding author on reasonable request.

Ethics approval and consent to participate

The horses were cared for according to accepted veterinary practices. The study was approved by the State Office for Consumer Protection and Food Safety (LAVES) in accordance with the German Animal Welfare Law (case number: 33.8–42502-04-17/2646).

Consent for publication

Not applicable.

Competing interests

The authors declare that they have no competing interests.

Author details

[1]Clinic for Horses, University of Veterinary Medicine Hannover, Foundation, Bünteweg 9, 30559 Hanover, Germany. [2]Institute of Animal Science, Faculty of Agricultural Sciences, University of Hohenheim, Fruwirthstraße 35, 70593 Stuttgart, Germany.

Received: 24 January 2020 Accepted: 4 May 2020
Published online: 24 May 2020

References

1. Jeffcott LB, Field JR, McLean JG, O'Dea K. Glucose tolerance and insulin sensitivity in ponies and Standardbred horses. Equine Vet J. 1986;18:97–101.
2. Field J, Jeffcott L. Equine laminits — another hypothesis for pathogenesis. Med Hypotheses. 1989;30:203–10.
3. Johnson PJ. The equine metabolic syndrome peripheral Cushing's syndrome. Vet Clin North Am Equine Pr. 2002;18:271–93.
4. Frank N, Geor RJJ, Bailey SRR, Durham AEE, Johnson PJJ, American College of Veterinary Internal M. Equine metabolic syndrome. J Vet Intern Med. 2010;24:467–75.
5. Durham AE, Frank N, McGowan CM, Menzies-Gow NJ, Roelfsema E, Vervuert I, et al. ECEIM consensus statement on equine metabolic syndrome. J Vet Intern Med. 2019;33:335–49.
6. Asplin KE, Sillence MN, Pollitt CC, McGowan CM. Induction of laminitis by prolonged hyperinsulinaemia in clinically normal ponies. Vet J. 2007;174:530–5.
7. de Laat M, Mc Gowan CM, Sillence MN, Pollitt CC. Equine laminitis: induced by 48 h hyperinsulinaemia in Standardbred horses. Equine Vet J. 2010;42:129–35.
8. Geor RJ, Harris P. Dietary Management of Obesity and Insulin Resistance: countering risk for laminitis. Vet Clin North Am - Equine Pract. 2009;25:51–65.
9. Carter RA, McCutcheon LJ, Valle E, Meilahn EN, Geor RJ. Effects of exercise training on adiposity, insulin sensitivity, and plasma hormone and lipid concentrations in overweight or obese, insulin-resistant horses. Am J Vet Res. 2010;71:314–21.
10. de Laat MA, Hampson BA, Sillence MN, Pollitt CC. Sustained, low-intensity exercise achieved by a dynamic feeding system decreases body fat in ponies. J Vet Intern Med. 2016;30:1732–8.
11. Van Weyenberg S, Hesta M, Buyse J, Janssens GPJ. The effect of weight loss by energy restriction on metabolic profile and glucose tolerance in ponies. J Anim Physiol Anim Nutr (Berl). 2008;92:538–45.
12. Dugdale AHA, Curtis GC, Cripps P, Harris PA, Argo MM. Effect of dietary restriction on body condition, composition and welfare of overweight and obese pony mares. Equine Vet J. 2010;42:600–10.
13. Argo CMCG, Curtis GC, Grove-White D, Dugdale AHA, Barfoot CF, Harris PA. Weight loss resistance: a further consideration for the nutritional management of obese Equidae. Vet J. 2012;194:179–88.
14. Gill JC, Pratt-Phillips SE, Mansmann R, Siciliano PD. Weight loss Management in Client-Owned Horses. J Equine Vet Sci. 2016;39:80–9.
15. Bamford NJ, Potter SJ, Baskerville CL, Harris PA, Bailey SR. Influence of dietary restriction and low-intensity exercise on weight loss and insulin sensitivity in obese equids. J Vet Intern Med. 2019;33:280–6.
16. Ungru J, Blüher M, Coenen M, Raila J, Boston R, Vervuert I. Effects of body weight reduction on blood adipokines and subcutaneous adipose tissue adipokine mRNA expression profiles in obese ponies. Vet Rec. 2012;171:528.
17. Morgan RA, Keen JA, McGowan CM. Treatment of equine metabolic syndrome: a clinical case series. Equine Vet J. 2016;48:422–6.
18. Bamford NJ, Potter SJ, Harris PA, Bailey SR. Effect of increased adiposity on insulin sensitivity and adipokine concentrations in horses and ponies fed a high-fat diet, with or without a once daily high-glycaemic meal. Equine Vet J. 2016;48:399–404.
19. Frank N, Tadros EM. Insulin dysregulation. Equine Vet J. 2014;46:103–12.
20. de Laat MA, McGree JM, Sillence MN. Equine hyperinsulinemia: investigation of the enteroinsular axis during insulin dysregulation. Am J Physiol - Endocrinol Metab. 2015;310:ajpendo.00362.2015.
21. Dühlmeier R, Deegen E, Fuhrmann H, Widdel A, Sallmann HP, Duhlmeier R, et al. Glucose-dependent insulinotropic polypeptide (GIP) and the enteroinsular axis in equines (Equus caballus). Comp Biochem Physiol A Mol Integr Physiol. 2001;129:563–75.
22. Lerner RL, Porte D. Relationships between intravenous glucose loads, insulin responses and glucose disappearance rate. J Clin Endocrinol Metab. 1971;33:409–17.
23. Dugdale AH, Grove-White D, Curtis GC, Harris PA, Argo CM. Body condition scoring as a predictor of body fat in horses and ponies. Vet J. 2012;194:173–8.
24. Jansson A, Stefansdottir G, Torres JCR, Ragnarsson S. Plasma insulin concentration is affected by body condition in Icelandic horses. Acta Vet Scand. 2015;57:2015.
25. Murphy D, Reid SW, Love S. The effect of age and diet on the oral glucose tolerance test in ponies. Equine Vet J. 1997;29:467–70.
26. Hart KA, Wochele DM, Norton NA, Mcfarlane D, Wooldridge AA, Frank N. Effect of age, season, body condition, and endocrine status on serum free cortisol fraction and insulin concentration in horses. J Vet Intern Med. 2016;30:653–63.
27. Moore JL, Siciliano PD, Pratt-Phillips SE. Voluntary energy intake and expenditure in obese and lean horses consuming ad libitum forage. J Equine Vet Sci. 2019;74:13–20.
28. Lindase SS, Nostell KE, Muller CE, Jensen-Waern M, Brojer JT. Effects of diet-induced weight gain and turnout to pasture on insulin sensitivity in moderately insulin resistant horses. Am J Vet Res. 2016;77:300–9.
29. Jacob SI, Geor RJ, Weber PSD, Harris PA, McCue ME. Effect of age and dietary carbohydrate profiles on glucose and insulin dynamics in horses. Equine Vet J. 2017;38:42–9.
30. Pratt SE, Geor RJ, Mccutcheon LJ. Effects of dietary energy source and physical conditioning on insulin sensitivity and glucose tolerance in Standardbred horses. Equine Vet J. 2006;38:579–84.
31. Argo CMG, Dugdale AHA, McGowan CM. Considerations for the use of restricted, soaked grass hay diets to promote weight loss in the management of equine metabolic syndrome and obesity. Vet J. 2015;206:170–7.
32. Bird SR, Hawley JA. Update on the effects of physical activity on insulin sensitivity in humans. BMJ Open Sport Exerc Med. 2017;2:1–26.
33. de Sousa MV, Fukui R, Krustrup P, Pereira RMR, Silva PRS, Rodrigues AC, et al. Positive effects of football on fitness, lipid profile, and insulin resistance in Brazilian patients with type 2 diabetes. Scand J Med Sci Sports. 2014;24:57–65.

34. Stuart CA, South MA, Lee ML, McCurry MP, Howell MEAA, Ramsey MW, et al. Insulin responsiveness in metabolic syndrome after eight weeks of cycle training. Med Sci Sports Exerc. 2013;45:2021–9.
35. Trussardi Fayh AP, Lopes AL, Fernandes PR, Reischak-Oliveira A, Friedman R. Impact of weight loss with or without exercise on abdominal fat and insulin resistance in obese individuals: a randomised clinical trial. Br J Nutr. 2013; 110:486–92.
36. Fitzgerald DM, Walsh DM, Sillence MN, Pollitt CC, de Laat MA. Insulin and incretin responses to grazing in insulin-dysregulated and healthy ponies. J Vet Intern Med. 2018;33:225–32.
37. Wyse CA, McNie KA, Tannahill VJ, Love S, Murray JK, Tannahil VJ, et al. Prevalence of obesity in riding horses in Scotland. Vet Rec. 2008;162:590–1.
38. Meier ADD, de Laat MAA, Reiche DBB, Pollitt CCC, Walsh DMM, McGree JMM, et al. The oral glucose test predicts laminitis risk in ponies fed a diet high in nonstructural carbohydrates. Domest Anim Endocrinol. 2018;63:1–9.
39. Warnken T, Schumacher S, Schmidt P, Huber K, Feige K. The impact of different glucose dosages in Oral glucose test for assessment of insulin Dysregulation. J Vet Intern Med. 2018;32:2144–309.
40. Warnken T, Huber K, Feige K. Comparison of three different methods for the quantification of equine insulin. BMC Vet Res. 2016;12:196.
41. R Core Team. R: A Language and Environment for Statistical Computing 2019.
42. Singmann H, Bolker B, Westfall J, Aust F. afex: analysis of factorial experiments; 2019.
43. Pinheiro J, Bates D, DebRoy S, Sarkar D, R Core Team. nlme: linear and nonlinear mixed effects models n.d.
44. Lenth R. emmeans: estimated marginal means, aka least-squares means; 2019.

Publisher's Note

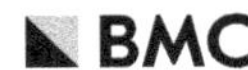

4. Manuscript 3

Metabolic impact of weight variations in Icelandic horses

Julien Delarocque[1]*, Florian Frers[1], Korinna Huber[2], Klaus Jung[3], Karsten Feige[1], Tobias Warnken[1]

[1] Clinic for Horses, University of Veterinary Medicine Hannover, Foundation, Hannover, Germany.

[2] Institute of Animal Science, Faculty of Agricultural Sciences, University of Hohenheim, Stuttgart, Germany.

[3] Institute for Animal Breeding and Genetics, University of Veterinary Medicine Hannover, Foundation, Hannover, Germany.

* Corresponding author

State of publication:

Published in PeerJ 9:e10764
DOI: 10.7717/peerj.10764

Contributions to the manuscript:

T. Warnken, K. Feige and J. Delarocque designed the experiments. J. Delarocque performed the experiments. J. Delarocque measured the insulin concentrations, prepared the figures, and wrote the paper. J. Delarocque analysed the data. All authors contributed to the interpretation of the results, reviewed drafts of the paper, and accepted the final manuscript.

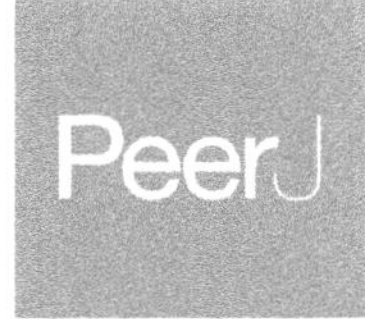

Metabolic impact of weight variations in Icelandic horses

Julien Delarocque[1], Florian Frers[1], Korinna Huber[2], Klaus Jung[3], Karsten Feige[1] and Tobias Warnken[1]

[1] Clinic for Horses, University of Veterinary Medicine Hannover, Foundation, Hannover, Germany
[2] Institute of Animal Science, Faculty of Agricultural Sciences, Universität Hohenheim, Stuttgart, Germany
[3] Institute for Animal Breeding and Genetics, Tierärztliche Hochschule Hannover, Hannover, Germany

ABSTRACT

Background. Insulin dysregulation (ID) is an equine endocrine disorder, which is often accompanied by obesity and various metabolic perturbations. The relationship between weight variations and fluctuations of the insulin response to oral glucose tests (OGT) as well as the metabolic impact of ID have been described previously. The present study seeks to characterize the concomitant metabolic impact of variations in the insulin response and bodyweight during repeated OGTs using a metabolomics approach.
Methods. Nineteen Icelandic horses were subjected to five OGTs over one year and their bodyweight, insulin and metabolic response were monitored. Analysis of metabolite concentrations depending on time (during the OGT), relative bodyweight (rWeight; defined as the bodyweight at one OGT divided by the mean bodyweight across all OGTs) and relative insulin response ($rAUC_{ins}$; defined accordingly from the area under the insulin curve during OGT) was performed using linear models. Additionally, the pathways significantly associated with time, rWeight and $rAUC_{ins}$ were identified by rotation set testing.
Results. The results suggested that weight gain and worsening of ID activate distinct metabolic pathways. The metabolic profile associated with weight gain indicated an increased activation of arginase, while the pathways associated with time and $rAUC_{ins}$ were consistent with the expected effect of glucose and insulin, respectively. Overall, more metabolites were significantly associated with rWeight than with $rAUC_{ins}$.

Submitted 8 September 2020
Accepted 22 December 2020
Published 28 January 2021

Corresponding author
Julien Delarocque,
julien.delarocque@tiho-hannover.de

Academic editor
Mohammed Gagaoua

Additional Information and Declarations can be found on page 11

DOI 10.7717/peerj.10764

Subjects Biochemistry, Veterinary Medicine, Zoology
Keywords Equine metabolic syndrome, Insulin dysregulation, Oral glucose test, Obesity, Metabolomics, Pathway analysis

INTRODUCTION

Insulin dysregulation (ID) is an equine endocrine disorder encompassing insulin resistance (IR) and basal or post-prandial hyperinsulinemia (HI), which predisposes horses for a crippling hoof condition called laminitis (*Frank & Tadros, 2014*). The oral glucose test (OGT) can be used to diagnose and quantify ID as it seizes both its enteric and systemic component (*De Laat, McGree & Sillence, 2015*; *Bertin & Laat, 2017*).

The impact of weight gain or weight loss on IR and ID has been described numerous times (*Van Weyenberg et al., 2008*; *Carter et al., 2009*; *Morgan, Keen & McGowan, 2016*; *Bamford et al., 2019*), substantiating obesity as a major risk factor for ID (*Geor & Harris, 2009*; *Morgan, McGowan & Mcgowan, 2014*) and establishing dietary energy restrictions and exercise programs as main requirements for the management of patients with this condition (Durham et al., 2019).

Because of its central role in energy metabolism, insulin is tied to many molecule classes. For example, amino acids have long been known to exert a regulatory function on β-cells and increase insulin secretion whereas insulin regulates protein synthesis (Floyd et al., 1966; Felig, 1975; Kimball, Vary & Jefferson, 1994). Some amino acids and derived biogenic amines or even broader classes of lipids (e.g., phosphatidylcholines, lysophosphatidylcholines and sphingomyelins) have been associated with specific pathomechanisms of metabolic conditions (Newsholme et al., 2007; Holland et al., 2008; McKnight et al., 2010). Therefore, metabolomics approaches covering this broad range of molecules have been used for the identification of candidate biomarkers and to investigate the pathophysiology of such conditions or their risk factors (Pallares-Méndez et al., 2016; Lent-Schochet et al., 2019). In contrast to hypothesis-driven approaches, such high-throughput methods aim to describe the studied systems in a global way, including their often complex interactions and capable of discovering unmapped pathways (Kell & Oliver, 2004).

Similar methods have been used in horses with ID, suggesting, for example, an impact of ID on the tricarboxylic acid cycle (Jacob et al., 2018). Previous experiments using the same assay were successful in identifying potential biomarkers of ID but did not include predictors related to bodyweight (Kenéz Warnken, Feige & Huber, 2018; Delarocque et al., 2020b). Besides the effect of weight gain on the lipidome (Blaue et al., 2019; Coleman et al., 2019), little is known about the relationship between obesity and the metabolome in horses. Since the relationship between variations in body weight and IR or ID is well known, an impact of such variations on the metabolites affected by ID is likely. The description of the respectively affected pathways could lead to new hypotheses for the treatment of these conditions. As a result, the objective of this retrospective study was to investigate the interplay between weight variations and changes in the insulin and metabolic response to repeated OGTs in an inductive framework. The main hypothesis was that weight gain and worsening of ID have a distinct metabolic impact during OGT.

MATERIALS & METHODS

The data presented here were obtained from blood samples collected as part of a study describing the relationship between weight variations and insulin response to an OGT (Delarocque et al., 2020a). The study was approved by the State Office for Consumer Protection and Food Safety (LAVES) in accordance with the German Animal Welfare Law (File #33.8–42502–04-17/2646).

Horses

Nineteen university-owned Icelandic horses of mixed metabolic status from two herds were enrolled in this project. One group included five horses (1 stallion, 4 geldings; median age: 17 years, range: 9–17 years), while the other comprised fourteen horses (11 mares, 3 geldings; median age: 21 years, range: 14–29 years). Both groups had access to neighboring pastures and were fed hay from the same batches.

Oral glucose tests

Five OGT were conducted at even intervals over one year. The horses were weighed using a mobile weighing scale (accuracy: 1%, resolution: 1 kg, precision: 2 kg) 9 to 16 days prior to each test. The horses were fasted for 12 h. In the morning (8:00–9:00 a.m.), a jugular vein catheter was aseptically placed for blood collection. After a basal blood sample had been drawn, 0.5 g/kg bwt glucose was administered *via* a nasogastric tube. Further blood samples were collected 30, 60, 120, 180 and 240 min later. After collection, the samples were separated into potassium EDTA and Z serum clot activator vacuum tubes (Greiner Bio-One International GmbH, Frickenhausen, Germany). The EDTA tubes were chilled at 4 °C, while the serum tubes were left to clot at room temperature. They were centrifuged at 4,000 g for 10 min within 6 h, for the plasma and serum supernatants to be collected, aliquoted and stored at –80 °C until further analysis.

Insulin measurements

Serum insulin concentrations were measured in duplicate at the end of the experimental phase using an equine-optimized ELISA (Mercodia Equine Insulin ELISA; Mercodia AB, Sylveniusgatan 8A, Uppsala, Sweden; inter-assay coefficient of variation: 7.7%) previously validated for use in horses.

Metabolomic assay

Metabolomic profiling of the 0 and 120 min plasma samples was performed at the Fraunhofer Institute of Toxicology and Experimental Medicine ITEM, Hanover, Germany, using the AbsoluteIDQ p180 Kit (Biocrates life sciences AG, Innsbruck, Austria). This assay includes up to 188 metabolites related to glycolysis, oxidative processes, lipid degradation and inflammatory signaling. Amino acids and biogenic amines were measured by liquid chromatography-tandem mass spectrometry while acylcarnitines, hexoses, phosphatidylcholines (PCs), lysophosphatidylcholines (LysoPCs) and sphingomyelins (SMs) were quantified using flow injection analysis-tandem mass spectrometry.

Statistical analysis

Statistical analysis was performed with R 4.0.0 (*R Core Team, 2020*). Metabolites with over 50% of values below the limit of detection were discarded. Remaining values below limit of detection were set to limit of detection/2. Missing values were imputed by the k-nearest neighbors method (*Hastie et al., 1999*). Measurement batches were aligned using the QC-RLSC method (*Dunn et al., 2011*). Metabolites with a coefficient of variation over 20% within the quality control samples were removed from further analysis. Substance class summaries of metabolite concentrations and the kynurenine to tryptophan ratio were computed. Values were then $\log_2$-transformed, adjusted for measurement and experimental (OGT replicates) batches using the 'removeBatchEffect' function from the 'limma' package (*Ritchie et al., 2015*), auto-scaled and quantile-normalized (*Bolstad et al., 2003*).

The relative weight (rWeight; weight at one OGT divided by the mean weight across all OGTs) and relative area under the insulin curve over time ($rAUC_{ins}$; defined similarly) were used as predictors of metabolite concentrations alongside the time of the OGT in a mixed linear model adjusted for group, age and sex using the 'limma' package to investigate the metabolic impact of weight variations and the insulin response.

Metabolite set enrichment analysis (MSEA) was performed using the 'mroast' function from the 'limma' package. According to the definition of Goeman & Bühlmann (2007), this function provides a self-contained set test relying on the principle of rotation applicable to linear models (Wu et al., 2010). Metabolite identifiers were obtained from the human metabolome database (Wishart et al., 2018) and associated with metabolic pathway identifiers from the small molecule pathway database (Jewison et al., 2014). Long-chain phospholipid concentrations in the p180 assay can represent the sum of several physiologically close isomers. In such cases, the first best match from the human metabolome database was kept as a metabolite identifier. Only pathways including at least three distinct metabolites from the cleaned dataset were kept for analysis.

P-values were adjusted for multiple comparisons using the method of Benjamini–Hochberg (Benjamini & Hochberg, 1995). Statistical significance was set at 0.05 (after adjustment for multiplicity).

RESULTS

Clinical parameters

The evolution of the insulin response to the OGT and bodyweight during the study period was described previously (Delarocque et al., 2020a). Briefly, the variations in bodyweight were similar in both groups with an overall median maximal weight difference of 43 kg (11%) while the variations in the insulin response differed. On the small pasture a median maximal variation of the AUC_{ins} of 68% was observed, while horses on the large pasture had a median maximal variation of 123%.

Despite a general trend of weight loss over the study period, the horses gained weight between two successive OGTs in 29% of the cases. The insulin response and bodyweight of the horses at each OGT are provided as an additional file (Table S1).

None of the horses developed laminitis or showed any other clinical abnormalities throughout the study.

Data preparation

Substance class summaries and the kynurenine/tryptophan ratio were added to the 188 metabolites measured by the Biocrates AbsoluteIDQ p180 Kit, resulting in 194 features. After preprocessing, 116 features were still present, as summarized in Table 1.

Nineteen horses were each subjected to five OGTs, for each of which two timepoints were considered in the metabolome, resulting in 190 samples.

Linear models

The impact of the time during the OGT, rWeight and $rAUC_{ins}$ on the metabolite concentrations was investigated using linear models. The first factor describes the time course of metabolite concentrations during the OGT, the second one represents the impact of variations in bodyweight and the third one shows the influence of changes in the insulin response.

Table 1 **Metabolites available before and after data pre-processing.** Summarized values are the sums of plasma concentrations of metabolites by groups (e.g., sum of acylcarnitines) or ratios like the kynurenine:tryptohphan-ratio, which is of interest in the scope of inflammatory processes.

Class	Before pre-processing	After pre-processing
Acylcarnitines	40	1
Amino acids	21	20
Biogenic amines	21	11
Glycerophospholipids	90	65
Sphingolipids	15	13
Sugars	1	1
Summarized values	6	5
Total	194	116

The number of metabolites significantly associated with each of the factors of interest from the linear model are displayed in Fig. 1. The greatest number of metabolites was associated with rWeight, followed by the effect of time during the OGT. Many metabolites were affected by more than one of these factors but not necessarily in the same direction (i.e., a metabolite might have been negatively associated with rWeight and positively associated with $rAUC_{ins}$, as shown in Fig. 2). The five metabolites affected by all three factors were arginine (Arg), serine (Ser) and the PCs: PC aa C32:1, PC aa C34:3 and PC aa C34:4. Most of the metabolites affected by both rWeight and time were PCs as well. The sum of hexoses is essentially representative of glucose during the OGT and was positively associated with$rAUC_{ins}$ and time.

Figure 2 visualizes the metabolic impact of rWeight (A) and $rAUC_{ins}$ (B) at each time point using heatmaps. While all metabolites significantly associated with $rAUC_{ins}$ are shown (Fig. 2B), only the top 20 metabolites significantly associated with rWeight are presented (Fig. 2A). Overall, the same patterns are visible at 0 and 120 min, however, the gradient was more pronounced at one of the timepoints for some metabolites (e.g., ornithine (Orn) concentrations increased with rWeight at both timepoints, however, this was more pronounced before oral glucose loading [0 min]). The metabolites predominantly affected were glycerophospholipids. The effect of $rAUC_{ins}$ on this class was exclusively negative and partly opposite to the effect rWeight (e.g., PC aa C36:5). It should be noted that the fold changes, indicating the changes in normalized metabolite concentrations for each unit of rWeight of $rAUC_{ins}$, cannot be directly compared since they are on different scales.

Asymmetric dimethylarginine (ADMA) was negatively associated with $rAUC_{ins}$. By contrast, the amino acids arginine, serine and alanine (Ala) were positively correlated with this factor. Interestingly, arginine displayed a negative association with rWeight, alongside phenylalanine (Phe), trans-4-hydroxyproline (t4-OH-Pro) and four SMs.

Metabolite set enrichment analysis

Seventeen pathways contained three or more metabolites and were available for MSEA. As presented in Fig. 3, all pathways were significantly, mostly negatively, associated with the effect of time in the OGT. While all pathways were significantly associated with rWeight as well, this effect is more ambiguous, with fewer pathways displaying an obvious positive

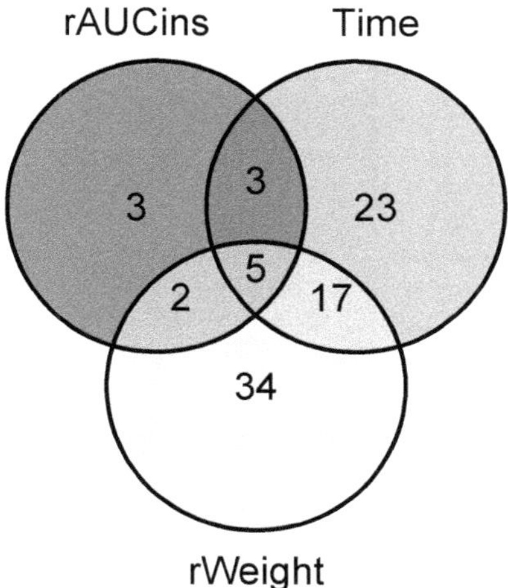

Figure 1 **Venn diagram of the metabolites significantly associated with the factors of interest in the linear model.** Each circle represents one factor of interest. The number within each region stands for the numbers of metabolites significantly associated with one or more of these factors according to the circles overlapping. As an example, two metabolites were significantly associated with both $rAUC_{ins}$ and rWeight, although the direction of association can vary (positive or negative).

Full-size DOI: 10.7717/peerj.10764/fig-1

or negative association. Nevertheless, the metabolism of alanine, glutamate, histidine and purine appeared to be positively associated with rWeight (i.e., more active upon weight gain). As for $rAUC_{ins}$, it had a positive impact on metabolites from the glucose-alanine and urea cycle and a pattern compatible with the Warburg effect. Overall, the effect of rWeight and $rAUC_{ins}$ were opposed to the effect of time.

DISCUSSION

The metabolic response of 19 horses to five OGTs was investigated while considering the impact of changes in bodyweight and the insulin response. The underlying aim was to illustrate and distinguish the impact of weight gain and an aggravation of ID on the metabolism. Univariate analysis highlighted the impact of these effects on glycerophospholipids. The effects of the relative weight and insulin response in MSEA were opposed to the effect of time in the OGT, which describes the immediate metabolic response induced by the glucose bolus.

Metabolic impact of variations in bodyweight

Variations in bodyweight were represented by the rWeight, which allowed one to compare the evolution of bodyweight between horses. Positive associations between metabolite

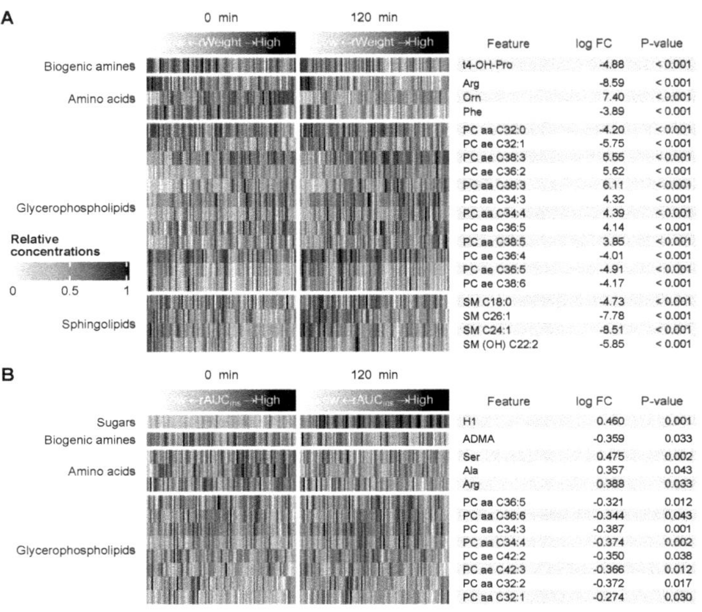

Figure 2 **Heatmaps of the metabolite concentrations significantly associated with rWeight (A) and $rAUC_{ins}$ (B).** Only the top 20 metabolites are shown for rWeight. The samples are arranged by increasing rWeight or $rAUC_{ins}$ and grouped by the time point of the OGT. This allows one to observe if the impact of the variables of interest is the same at both time points and prevents the effect of rWeight or $rAUC_{ins}$ to be masked by the effect of time (e.g., as would be the case for sugars [H1]).

Full-size DOI: 10.7717/peerj.10764/fig-2

concentrations and the rWeight can be interpreted as the metabolic impact of weight gain irrespective of its cause (the same being true for negative associations and weight loss). The quality of feed inducing weight gain affects the extent of ID (Bamford et al., 2016). Moreover, weight loss achieved by dietary restrictions and exercise can provide additional metabolic benefits compared to dietary restrictions alone (Carter et al., 2010; Moore, Siciliano & Pratt-Phillips, 2019; Bamford et al., 2019). Because physical activity energy expenditure and energy intake were not measured, the effect attributed to weight gain or loss in this retrospective study can result from any or both components. Additionally, the metabolic response to the OGT may vary depending on the proportions of metabolically active tissues (e.g., muscle mass *versus* adipose tissue) and their functional integrity (e.g., adipose tissue dysfunction). Neither parameter was assessed in the present study, but both might be affected by variations in bodyweight (Blaue et al., 2019; Reynolds et al., 2019).

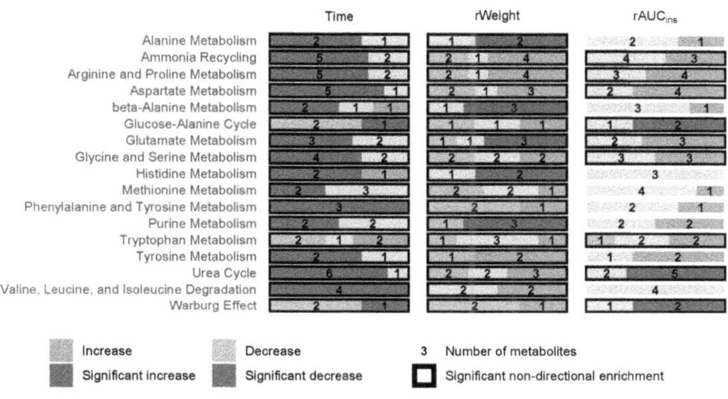

Figure 3 **Impact of the three factors of interest from the linear model on the 17 pathways included in MSEA.** Time is mostly associated with a decrease in metabolic activity, while the other two factors counterbalance this effect.

Full-size DOI: 10.7717/peerj.10764/fig-3

The metabolites PC aa C32:0, PC ae C36:2, PC ae C36:4, PC ae C36:5 and PC ae C38:6 have been previously reported to be negatively associated with the body mass index in humans (*Wallace et al., 2014*), while the metabolites SM C18:0, SM (OH) C22:2, t4-OH-Pro and SM C26:1 were decreased in type 2 diabetes mellitus (*Allalou et al., 2016*; *Isherwood et al., 2017*), showing good agreement with the results from the present study. It should be noted that the studies on diabetes mellitus included individuals with a mean body mass index over 30 or a higher mean body mass index in the diabetes group, which was compared to an obese/overweight group, so that a contribution of obesity to the effects observed is possible. Nevertheless, opposite patterns were also described for PC ae C36:2 (*Wallace et al., 2014*) and SM C18:0 (*Hanamatsu et al., 2014*). Overall, the similarity of the metabolites associated with obesity in humans and horses suggests the presence of common pathophysiological processes across species.

Decreased t4-OH-Pro has previously been associated with ID in horses (*Kenéz Warnken, Feige & Huber, 2018*), however, the impact of obesity was not analyzed. Since obesity is a major risk factor for ID, the present results appear to be compatible with the previous findings. Since proline hydroxylation requires the antioxidant ascorbic acid, it was hypothesized that hydroxyproline is an indirect marker of oxidative stress in several species (*Kenéz Warnken, Feige & Huber, 2018*; *Lent-Schochet et al., 2019*; *Zhang et al., 2020*). In addition to indicating oxidative stress, a decrease of t4-OH-Pro upon weight gain might arise from a lack of ascorbic acid secondarily to oxidative processes and result in the production of structurally unstable collagen, which could weaken the lamellar basement membrane. On the other hand, there is contradictory evidence regarding the association of HI or obesity and oxidative stress (Treiber et al., 2009; Pleasant et al., 2013; Banse et al., 2015).

The alanine metabolism was positively associated with weight gain, however alanine itself was not, so that the remaining metabolites are more representative of purine or, more probably, glutamate metabolism. Both glutamate and glutamate metabolism were significantly associated with rWeight. Monosodium l-glutamate was shown to suppress weight gain in rats, possibly by increasing the energy expenditure (Kondoh & Torii, 2008). Moreover, it was reported to increase satiety and reduce voluntary energy intake in humans (Kondoh & Torii, 2008). Therefore, the present findings could indicate a regulatory effect of glutamate metabolism upon weight gain.

Similarly, the impact of rWeight on beta-alanine and histidine metabolism, mainly mediated by glutamate, histidine and carnosine, might result from an adaptation to an increased lipogenesis (Mong, Chao & Yin, 2011).

Variations in arginine concentrations are attributable to its metabolization (among others into nitric oxide (NO), creatinine, ornithine and citrulline), the level of protein synthesis and turnover, de novo synthesis and dietary uptake (Morris, 2016). Nevertheless, based on the present results, it cannot be determined which mechanisms are associated with rWeight and $rAUC_{ins}$, respectively, or if these mechanisms are a cause or a consequence of ID or weight gain. Arginine has a potent vasodilatory effect mediated by NO (Bode-Böger, 2006). Therefore, it is interesting that vascular dysfunction has previously been associated with endocrinopathic laminitis (Morgan et al., 2016), which is the main clinical consequence of ID.

While arginine was strongly negatively associated with rWeight, the opposite was true for ornithine. This implies an inverse association between rWeight and the Arg:Orn ratio, which was reported to be negatively associated with arginase activity (Kashyap et al., 2008; Kövamees, Shemyakin & Pernow, 2016) since Arg is the immediate precursor of Orn in the arginase pathway (Morris, 2016). An increased arginase activity, which is supported by the present results, would result in competitive inhibition of NO synthetase, which could, in turn, affect endothelial function (Sourij et al., 2011).

Metabolic impact of changes in the insulin response

Changes in the insulin response were assessed using the $rAUC_{ins}$, which is the total insulin response approximated by the area under the insulin curve during the OGT (AUC_{ins}), relative to the horse's mean total insulin response. This measure makes the evolution of the insulin response comparable across horses. An increase in $rAUC_{ins}$ indicates a worsening of ID.

Arginine was positively associated with an increased insulin response ($\log_2$ fold-change $= 0.39$); however, in absolute numbers, this relationship was much weaker than the negative relationship between rWeight and arginine ($\log_2$ fold-change $= -8.59$). While the scales of rWeight and $rAUC_{ins}$ differ, the difference between the absolute fold changes remains obvious even when adjusted for the relationship reported previously between rWeight and $rAUC_{ins}$, where the impact of rWeight on $rAUC_{ins}$ was fivefold (Delarocque et al., 2020a). As weight gain is often associated with an aggravation of ID (Carter et al., 2010), the impact of rWeight on arginine might prevail on the effect of $rAUC_{ins}$ when only one of these measures is accounted for in the statistical model. Conversely, this result highlights that different metabolic mechanisms appear to be triggered by weight gain and worsening of ID.

Arginine is also known as an insulin secretagogue (*Floyd et al., 1966*), which might explain why arginine was positively associated with $rAUC_{ins}$ and negatively associated with rWeight.

The $rAUC_{ins}$ was also negatively associated with ADMA. However, the relevance for the pathomechanism of ID or laminitis remains unknown as this molecule inhibits nitric oxide synthesis (*Bode-Böger, 2006*).

The opposite impact of time and $rAUC_{ins}$ on the urea cycle is consistent with previous reports (*Hamberg & Vilstrup, 1994*). As expected, the induced hyperglycemia is associated with a decrease in products of the urea cycle, while HI is not. The positive effect of $rAUC_{ins}$ on urea cycle metabolites might be mediated by a reduction of hyperglycemia, which would imply an adequate insulin sensitivity of the liver even in insulin dysregulated horses.

Considerations on data analysis

Although rWeight has previously been reported to be linearly associated with $rAUC_{ins}$, it should be acknowledged that the correlation between the two was essentially conditional on the Group (see Methods/Animals) (*Delarocque et al., 2020a*). While the model was adjusted for the effect of Group, the predictors were not. The raw correlation between rWeight and $rAUC_{ins}$ was moderate ($r = 0.44$), but the coefficients associated with the predictors determined for each metabolite were barely affected by the exclusion of the other variable of interest from the model (Fig. S1). As a result, the model used in the present study does not appear to have been affected by collinearity.

It is necessary to map the metabolites to known pathways in order to perform MSEA. This presupposes sufficient knowledge of both the pathways and the metabolites, but this presumption is not fulfilled equally for all metabolites (in contrast to most genes). As an example, glycerophospholipids were largely impacted by both rWeight and $rAUC_{ins}$ but unrepresented in MSEA, which could represent a form of bias.

CONCLUSIONS

The results supported a pro-inflammatory impact of weight gain and suggested that it affects glutamate metabolism. The arginine concentrations were affected in opposite ways by rWeight and $rAUC_{ins}$, potentially inducing vascular dysfunction but also involved in the modulation of the insulin response. Both glutamate and arginine can easily be supplemented orally, warranting the exploration of new adjunct dietary approaches to hamper ID in future studies.

ACKNOWLEDGEMENTS

The authors thank Professor Wolfgang Leibold for his support and providing the horses and Dr Björn Steinbjörnsson for his help during the experiments and dedicated care to the horses.

ADDITIONAL INFORMATION AND DECLARATIONS

Funding

This publication was supported by Deutsche Forschungsgemeinschaft and University of Veterinary Medicine Hannover, Foundation within the funding programme Open Access Publishing. The funders had no role in study design, data collection and analysis, decision to publish, or preparation of the manuscript.

Grant Disclosures

The following grant information was disclosed by the authors:
Deutsche Forschungsgemeinschaft and University of Veterinary Medicine Hannover.

Competing Interests

The authors declare there are no competing interests.

Author Contributions

- Julien Delarocque conceived and designed the experiments, performed the experiments, analyzed the data, prepared figures and/or tables, authored or reviewed drafts of the paper, and approved the final draft.
- Florian Frers performed the experiments, authored or reviewed drafts of the paper, and approved the final draft.
- Korinna Huber and Klaus Jung analyzed the data, authored or reviewed drafts of the paper, and approved the final draft.
- Karsten Feige conceived and designed the experiments, analyzed the data, authored or reviewed drafts of the paper, and approved the final draft.
- Tobias Warnken conceived and designed the experiments, performed the experiments, authored or reviewed drafts of the paper, and approved the final draft.

Animal Ethics

The following information was supplied relating to ethical approvals (i.e., approving body and any reference numbers):

The study was approved by the State Office for Consumer Protection and Food Safety (LAVES)in accordance with the German Animal Welfare Law (33.8–42502–04-17/2646).

Data Availability

The following information was supplied regarding data availability:

Raw data is available in the Supplemental Files.

Supplemental Information

Supplemental information for this article can be found online at http://dx.doi.org/10.7717/peerj.10764#supplemental-information.

REFERENCES

Carter RA, McCutcheon LJ, George LA, Smith TL, Frank N, Geor RJ. 2009. Effects of diet-induced weight gain on insulin sensitivity and plasma hormone and lipid concentrations in horses. *American Journal of Veterinary Research* **70**:1250–1258 DOI 10.2460/ajvr.70.10.1250.

Allalou A, Nalla A, Prentice KJ, Liu Y, Zhang M, Dai FF, Ning X, Osborne LR, Cox BJ, Gunderson EP, Wheeler MB. 2016. A predictive metabolic signature for the transition from gestational diabetes mellitus to type 2 diabetes. *Diabetes* **65**:2529–2539 DOI 10.2337/db15-1720.

Bamford NJ, Potter SJ, Baskerville CL, Harris PA, Bailey SR. 2016. Effect of increased adiposity on insulin sensitivity and adipokine concentrations in different equine breeds adapted to cereal-rich or fat-rich meals. *The Veterinary Journal* **214**:14–20 DOI 10.1016/j.tvjl.2016.02.002.

Bamford NJ, Potter SJ, Baskerville CL, Harris PA, Bailey SR. 2019. Influence of dietary restriction and low-intensity exercise on weight loss and insulin sensitivity in obese equids. *Journal of Veterinary Internal Medicine* **33**:280–286 DOI 10.1111/jvim.15374.

Banse HE, Frank N, Kwong GPS, McFarlane D. 2015. Relationship of oxidative stress in skeletal muscle with obesity and obesity-associated hyperinsulinemia in horses. *Canadian Journal of Veterinary Research = Revue Canadienne de Recherche Veterinaire* **79**:329–338 DOI 10.1161/HYPERTENSIONAHA.110.164350.

Benjamini Y, Hochberg Y. 1995. Controlling the False Discovery Rate: A Practical and Powerful Approach to Multiple Testing. *Journal of the Royal Statistical Society. Series B (Methodological)* **57**:289–300 DOI 10.2307/2346101.

Bertin FR, De Laat MA. 2017. The diagnosis of equine insulin dysregulation. *Equine Veterinary Journal* **49**:570–576 DOI 10.1111/evj.12703.

Blaue D, Schedlbauer C, Starzonek J, Gittel C, Brehm W, Einspanier A, Vervuert I. 2019. Effects of body weight gain on insulin and lipid metabolism in equines. *Domestic Animal Endocrinology* **68**:111–118 DOI 10.1016/j.domaniend.2019.01.003.

Bode-Böger SM. 2006. Effect of L-arginine supplementation on NO production in man. *European Journal of Clinical Pharmacology* **62**:91–99 DOI 10.1007/s00228-005-0004-z.

Carter RA, McCutcheon LJ, Valle E, Meilahn EN, Geor RJ. 2010. Effects of exercise training on adiposity, insulin sensitivity, and plasma hormone and lipid concentrations in overweight or obese, insulin-resistant horses. *American Journal of Veterinary Research* **71**:314–321 DOI 10.2460/ajvr.71.3.314.

Coleman MC, Whitfield-Cargile CM, Madrigal RG, Cohen ND. 2019. Comparison of the microbiome, metabolome, and lipidome of obese and non-obese horses. *PLOS ONE* **14**:1–17 DOI 10.1371/journal.pone.0215918.

De Laat MA, McGree JM, Sillence MN. 2015. Equine hyperinsulinemia: investigation of the enteroinsular axis during insulin dysregulation. *American Journal of Physiology - Endocrinology And Metabolism* **310**:E61–E72 DOI 10.1152/ajpendo.00362.2015.

Delarocque J, Frers F, Huber K, Feige K, Warnken T. 2020a. Weight loss is linearly associated with a reduction of the insulin response to an oral glucose test in Icelandic horses. *BMC Veterinary Research* **16**:151 DOI 10.1186/s12917-020-02356-w.

Delarocque J, Frers F, Jung K, Warnken T, Feige K. 2020b. Metabolic changes induced by oral glucose tests in horses and their diagnostic use. *Journal of Veterinary Internal Medicine*. Epub ahead of print 2020 5 December DOI 10.1111/jvim.15992.

Dunn WB, Broadhurst D, Begley P, Zelena E, Francis-Mcintyre S, Anderson N, Brown M, Knowles JD, Halsall A, Haselden JN, Nicholls AW, Wilson ID, Kell DB, Goodacre R. 2011. Procedures for large-scale metabolic profiling of serum and plasma using gas chromatography and liquid chromatography coupled to mass spectrometry. *Nature Protocols* **6**:1060–1083 DOI 10.1038/nprot.2011.335.

Durham AE, Frank N, McGowan CM, Menzies-Gow NJ, Roelfsema E, Vervuert I, Feige K, Fey K. 2019. ECEIM consensus statement on equine metabolic syndrome. *Journal of Veterinary Internal Medicine* **33**:335–349 DOI 10.1111/jvim.15423.

Felig P. 1975. Amino acid metabolism in man. *Annual Review of Biochemistry* **44**:933–955 DOI 10.1146/annurev.bi.44.070175.004441.

Floyd JC, Fajans SS, Conn JW, Knopf RF, Rull J. 1966. Stimulation of insulin secretion by amino acids. *Journal of Clinical Investigation* **45**:1487–1502 DOI 10.1172/JCI105456.

Frank N, Tadros EM. 2014. Insulin dysregulation. *Equine Veterinary Journal* **46**:103–112 DOI 10.1111/evj.12169.

Geor RJ, Harris P. 2009. Dietary management of obesity and insulin resistance: countering risk for laminitis. *Veterinary Clinics of North America - Equine Practice* **25**:51–65 DOI 10.1016/j.cveq.2009.02.001.

Goeman JJ, Bühlmann P. 2007. Analyzing gene expression data in terms of gene sets: methodological issues. *Bioinformatics* **23**:980–987 DOI 10.1093/bioinformatics/btm051.

Hamberg O, Vilstrup H. 1994. Effects of insulin and glucose on urea synthesis in normal man, independent of pancreatic hormone secretion. *Journal of Hepatology* **21**:381–387 DOI 10.1016/S0168-8278(05)80317-4.

Hanamatsu H, Ohnishi S, Sakai S, Yuyama K, Mitsutake S, Takeda H, Hashino S, Igarashi Y. 2014. Altered levels of serum sphingomyelin and ceramide containing distinct acyl chains in young obese adults. *Nutrition and Diabetes* **4**:e141–7 DOI 10.1038/nutd.2014.38.

Hastie T, Tibshirani R, Sherlock G, Eisen M, Brown P, Botstein D. 1999. Imputing missing data for gene expression arrays.

Holland WL, Knotts TA, Chavez JA, Wang L-P, Hoehn KL, Summers SA. 2008. Lipid mediators of insulin resistance. *Nutrition Reviews* **65**:S39–S46 DOI 10.1111/j.1753-4887.2007.tb00327.x.

Bolstad BM, Irizarry R, Astrand M, Speed TP. 2003. A comparison of normalization methods for high density oligonucleotide array data based on variance and bias. *Bioinformatics* **19**:185–193 DOI 10.1093/bioinformatics/19.2.185.

Isherwood CM, Van der Veen DR, Johnston JD, Skene DJ. 2017. Twenty-four-hour rhythmicity of circulating metabolites: effect of body mass and type 2 diabetes. *FASEB Journal* **31**:5557–5567 DOI 10.1096/fj.201700323R.

Jacob SI, Murray KJ, Rendahl AK, Geor RJ, Schultz NE, McCue ME. 2018. Metabolic perturbations in Welsh Ponies with insulin dysregulation, obesity, and laminitis. *Journal of Veterinary Internal Medicine* **32**:1215–1233 DOI 10.1111/jvim.15095.

Jewison T, Su Y, Disfany FM, Liang Y, Knox C, MacIejewski A, Poelzer J, Huynh J, Zhou Y, Arndt D, Djoumbou Y, Liu Y, Deng L, Guo AC, Han B, Pon A, Wilson M, Rafatnia S, Liu P, Wishart DS. 2014. SMPDB 2.0: big improvements to the small molecule pathway database. *Nucleic Acids Research* **42**:478–484 DOI 10.1093/nar/gkt1067.

Kashyap SR, Lara A, Zhang R, Park YM, DeFronzo RA. 2008. Insulin reduces plasma arginase activity in type 2 diabetic patients. *Diabetes Care* **31**:134–139 DOI 10.2337/dc07-1198.

Kell DB, Oliver SG. 2004. Here is the evidence, now what is the hypothesis? The complementary roles of inductive and hypothesis-driven science in the post-genomic era. *BioEssays* **26**:99–105 DOI 10.1002/bies.10385.

Kenéz Warnken T, Feige K, Huber K. 2018. Lower plasma trans-4-hydroxyproline and methionine sulfoxide levels are associated with insulin dysregulation in horses. *BMC Veterinary Research* **14**:146 DOI 10.1186/s12917-018-1479-z.

Kimball SR, Vary TC, Jefferson LS. 1994. Regulation of protein synthesis by insulin. *Annual Review of Physiology* **56**:321–348 DOI 10.1146/annurev.ph.56.030194.001541.

Kondoh T, Torii K. 2008. MSG intake suppresses weight gain, fat deposition, and plasma leptin levels in male Sprague-Dawley rats. *Physiology and Behavior* **95**:135–144 DOI 10.1016/j.physbeh.2008.05.010.

Kövamees O, Shemyakin A, Pernow J. 2016. Amino acid metabolism reflecting arginase activity is increased in patients with type 2 diabetes and associated with endothelial dysfunction. *Diabetes and Vascular Disease Research* **13**:354–360 DOI 10.1177/1479164116643916.

Lent-Schochet D, McLaughlin M, Ramakrishnan N, Jialal I. 2019. Exploratory metabolomics of metabolic syndrome: a status report. *World Journal of Diabetes* **10**:23–36 DOI 10.4239/wjd.v10.i1.23.

McKnight JR, Satterfield MC, Jobgen WS, Smith SB, Spencer TE, Meininger CJ, McNeal CJ, Wu G. 2010. Beneficial effects of L-arginine on reducing obesity: potential mechanisms and important implications for human health. *Amino Acids* **39**:349–357 DOI 10.1007/s00726-010-0598-z.

Mong MC, Chao CY, Yin MC. 2011. Histidine and carnosine alleviated hepatic steatosis in mice consumed high saturated fat diet. *European Journal of Pharmacology* **653**:82–88 DOI 10.1016/j.ejphar.2010.12.001.

Moore JL, Siciliano PD, Pratt-Phillips SE. 2019. Effects of diet versus exercise on morphometric measurements, blood hormone concentrations, and oral sugar test response in obese horses. *Journal of Equine Veterinary Science* **78**:38–45 DOI 10.1016/j.jevs.2019.03.214.

Morgan RA, Keen JA, McGowan CM. 2016. Treatment of equine metabolic syndrome: a clinical case series. *Equine Veterinary Journal* **48**:422–426 DOI 10.1111/evj.12445.

Morgan RA, Keen JA, Walker BR, Hadoke PWF. 2016. Vascular dysfunction in horses with endocrinopathic laminitis. *PLOS ONE* **11**:1–14 DOI 10.1371/journal.pone.0163815.

Morgan RA, McGowan TW, Mcgowan CM. 2014. Prevalence and risk factors for hyperinsulinaemia in ponies in Queensland, Australia. *Australian Veterinary Journal* **92**:101–106 DOI 10.1111/avj.12159.

Morris SM. 2016. Arginine metabolism revisited. *Journal of Nutrition* **146**:2579S–2586S DOI 10.3945/jn.115.226621.

Newsholme P, Bender K, Kiely A, Brennan L. 2007. Amino acid metabolism, insulin secretion and diabetes. *Biochemical Society Transactions* **35**:1180–1186 DOI 10.1042/BST0351180.

Pallares-Méndez R, Aguilar-Salinas CA, Cruz-Bautista I, Del Bosque-Plata L. 2016. Metabolomics in diabetes, a review. *Annals of Medicine* **48**:89–102 DOI 10.3109/07853890.2015.1137630.

Pleasant RSS, Suagee JKK, Thatcher CDD, Elvinger F, Geor RJJ. 2013. Adiposity, plasma insulin, leptin, lipids, and oxidative stress in mature light breed horses. *Journal of Veterinary Internal Medicine* **27**:576–582 DOI 10.1111/jvim.12056.

R Core Team. 2020. R: a language and environment for statistical computing. Vienna, Austria: R Foundation for Statistical Computing. *Available at https://www.R-project.org/*.

Reynolds A, Keen JA, Fordham T, Morgan RA. 2019. Adipose tissue dysfunction in obese horses with equine metabolic syndrome. *Equine Veterinary Journal* **51**:760–766 DOI 10.1111/evj.13097.

Ritchie ME, Phipson B, Wu D, Hu Y, Law CW, Shi W, Smyth GK. 2015. limma powers differential expression analyses for RNA-sequencing and microarray studies. *Nucleic Acids Research* **43**:e47–e47 DOI 10.1093/nar/gkv007.

Sourij H, Meinitzer A, Pilz S, Grammer TB, Winkelmann BR, Boehm BO, März W. 2011. Arginine bioavailability ratios are associated with cardiovascular mortality in patients referred to coronary angiography. *Atherosclerosis* **218**:220–225 DOI 10.1016/j.atherosclerosis.2011.04.041.

Treiber K, Carter R, Gay L, Williams C, Geor R. 2009. Inflammatory and redox status of ponies with a history of pasture-associated laminitis. *Veterinary Immunology and Immunopathology* **129**:216–220 DOI 10.1016/j.vetimm.2008.11.004.

Van Weyenberg S, Hesta M, Buyse J, Janssens GPJ. 2008. The effect of weight loss by energy restriction on metabolic profile and glucose tolerance in ponies. *Journal of Animal Physiology and Animal Nutrition* **92**:538–545 DOI 10.1111/j.1439-0396.2007.00744.x.

Wallace M, Morris C, O'Grada CM, Ryan M, Dillon ET, Coleman E, Gibney ER, Gibney MJ, Roche HM, Brennan L. 2014. Relationship between the lipidome, inflammatory markers and insulin resistance. *Molecular BioSystems* **10**:1586–1595 DOI 10.1039/C3MB70529C.

Wishart DS, Feunang YD, Marcu A, Guo AC, Liang K, Vázquez-Fresno R, Sajed T, Johnson D, Li C, Karu N, Sayeeda Z, Lo E, Assempour N, Berjanskii M, Singhal S, Arndt D, Liang Y, Badran H, Grant J, Serra-Cayuela A, Liu Y, Mandal R, Neveu V, Pon A, Knox C, Wilson M, Manach C, Scalbert A. 2018. HMDB 4.0: The human metabolome database for 2018. *Nucleic Acids Research* **46**:D608–D617 DOI 10.1093/nar/gkx1089.

Wu D, Lim E, Vaillant F, Asselin-Labat ML, Visvader JE, Smyth GK. 2010. ROAST: rotation gene set tests for complex microarray experiments. *Bioinformatics* **26**:2176–2182 DOI 10.1093/bioinformatics/btq401.

Zhang G, Zwierzchowski G, Mandal R, Wishart DS, Ametaj BN. 2020. Serum metabolomics identifies metabolite panels that differentiate lame dairy cows from healthy ones. *Metabolomics* **16**:1–22 DOI 10.1007/s11306-020-01693-z.

Supporting information

Data S1 Full dataset including the raw and preprocessed metabolite concentrations. The sheets of the spreadsheet include the sample data, feature data and raw and preprocessed concentration data. Rows of the sample data correspond to columns in the concentration data sheets (rownames correspond to column names) and rows of the feature data sheet correspond to the rows of the concentration data sheets.

[Supplemental Data S1.xlsx]

Table S1 Insulin response and bodyweight of the horses at each OGT. This data was presented in a previous publication describing the relationship between the relative bodyweight (rWeight) and relative insulin response ($rAUC_{ins}$). The present manuscript seeks to correlate this data to the metabolic response to OGT and thereby to describe the interplay between these three variables.

Horse	OGT	Weight (kg)	rWeight	AUC (µIU*min/ml)	rAUC	Group	Sex	Age (years)
1	OGT-I	311	1,078	6310,797	1,110	1	female	29
1	OGT-II	300	1,040	8067,288	1,419	1	female	29
1	OGT-III	294	1,019	9075,494	1,596	1	female	29
1	OGT-IV	284	0,984	1508,799	0,265	1	female	29
1	OGT-V	254	0,880	3466,758	0,610	1	female	29
2	OGT-I	394	1,041	28218,024	0,929	1	female	19
2	OGT-II	392	1,035	40944,195	1,347	1	female	19
2	OGT-III	381	1,006	44993,175	1,481	1	female	19
2	OGT-IV	366	0,967	23069,280	0,759	1	female	19
2	OGT-V	360	0,951	14716,554	0,484	1	female	19
4	OGT-I	389	1,061	52297,500	1,252	1	gelding	18
4	OGT-II	371	1,012	72696,765	1,740	1	gelding	18
4	OGT-III	367	1,001	43470,930	1,041	1	gelding	18
4	OGT-IV	360	0,982	19609,199	0,469	1	gelding	18
4	OGT-V	346	0,944	20814,864	0,498	1	gelding	18
5	OGT-I	364	1,052	3064,913	0,644	1	gelding	14
5	OGT-II	364	1,052	8401,539	1,767	1	gelding	14
5	OGT-III	346	1,000	7270,367	1,529	1	gelding	14
5	OGT-IV	325	0,939	3719,466	0,782	1	gelding	14
5	OGT-V	331	0,957	1322,651	0,278	1	gelding	14
6	OGT-I	399	1,028	49555,620	1,241	1	female	24
6	OGT-II	378	0,974	43686,795	1,094	1	female	24
6	OGT-III	397	1,023	51870,360	1,299	1	female	24
6	OGT-IV	403	1,039	29374,965	0,736	1	female	24
6	OGT-V	363	0,936	25119,270	0,629	1	female	24
7	OGT-I	449	1,067	25701,431	1,380	1	gelding	22
7	OGT-II	419	0,995	19846,755	1,065	1	gelding	22
7	OGT-III	422	1,002	19120,532	1,026	1	gelding	22
7	OGT-IV	415	0,986	15981,693	0,858	1	gelding	22
7	OGT-V	400	0,950	12487,604	0,670	1	gelding	22
8	OGT-I	400	1,042	31929,945	1,859	1	female	20
8	OGT-II	395	1,029	7867,581	0,458	1	female	20
8	OGT-III	369	0,961	24802,755	1,444	1	female	20
8	OGT-IV	384	1,000	8422,743	0,490	1	female	20
8	OGT-V	372	0,969	12847,191	0,748	1	female	20
9	OGT-I	317	1,080	6708,576	1,201	1	female	20
9	OGT-II	304	1,035	5969,961	1,069	1	female	20
9	OGT-III	289	0,984	8320,964	1,490	1	female	20
9	OGT-IV	287	0,978	4103,196	0,735	1	female	20
9	OGT-V	271	0,923	2818,752	0,505	1	female	20
10	OGT-I	371	1,047	23111,724	1,007	1	female	25
10	OGT-II	352	0,994	13106,460	0,571	1	female	25
10	OGT-III	360	1,016	55609,080	2,423	1	female	25
10	OGT-IV	360	1,016	11668,512	0,508	1	female	25

10	OGT-V	328	0,926	11247,765	0,490	1	female	25
12	OGT-I	400	1,012	124546,995	1,167	1	female	19
12	OGT-II	390	0,987	123389,280	1,156	1	female	19
12	OGT-III	401	1,015	112333,800	1,052	1	female	19
12	OGT-IV	405	1,025	101382,915	0,950	1	female	19
12	OGT-V	380	0,962	72113,043	0,676	1	female	19
13	OGT-I	355	1,123	13157,715	1,226	1	female	24
13	OGT-II	328	1,038	21437,565	1,997	1	female	24
13	OGT-III	317	1,003	8286,300	0,772	1	female	24
13	OGT-IV	306	0,968	5978,721	0,557	1	female	24
13	OGT-V	274	0,867	4807,610	0,448	1	female	24
14	OGT-I	403	1,048	4940,391	0,729	1	female	17
14	OGT-II	406	1,056	15337,250	2,265	1	female	17
14	OGT-III	393	1,022	4534,229	0,669	1	female	17
14	OGT-IV	363	0,944	3093,792	0,457	1	female	17
14	OGT-V	357	0,929	5958,854	0,880	1	female	17
19	OGT-I	446	1,080	35880,560	1,619	1	female	22
19	OGT-II	423	1,025	20346,791	0,918	1	female	22
19	OGT-III	416	1,008	16506,720	0,745	1	female	22
19	OGT-IV	405	0,981	9720,429	0,438	1	female	22
19	OGT-V	374	0,906	28388,600	1,281	1	female	22
20	OGT-I	343	1,115	10604,415	1,518	1	female	25
20	OGT-II	323	1,050	9305,189	1,332	1	female	25
20	OGT-III	311	1,011	8291,370	1,187	1	female	25
20	OGT-IV	295	0,959	4270,188	0,611	1	female	25
20	OGT-V	266	0,865	2450,643	0,351	1	female	25
3	OGT-I	404	1,026	7030,824	0,735	2	stallion	14
3	OGT-II	418	1,061	17017,427	1,780	2	stallion	14
3	OGT-III	392	0,995	4949,886	0,518	2	stallion	14
3	OGT-IV	375	0,952	11324,139	1,184	2	stallion	14
3	OGT-V	380	0,965	7492,392	0,783	2	stallion	14
11	OGT-I	421	1,056	5636,367	0,413	2	gelding	17
11	OGT-II	421	1,056	18163,020	1,330	2	gelding	17
11	OGT-III	394	0,988	22791,030	1,669	2	gelding	17
11	OGT-IV	377	0,946	11200,505	0,820	2	gelding	17
11	OGT-V	380	0,953	10494,047	0,768	2	gelding	17
15	OGT-I	415	1,026	5964,333	0,602	2	gelding	9
15	OGT-II	425	1,051	10497,711	1,059	2	gelding	9
15	OGT-III	391	0,967	11931,572	1,204	2	gelding	9
15	OGT-IV	394	0,974	8428,136	0,851	2	gelding	9
15	OGT-V	397	0,982	12725,421	1,284	2	gelding	9
16	OGT-I	414	1,042	6109,598	0,818	2	gelding	17
16	OGT-II	413	1,039	7813,625	1,046	2	gelding	17
16	OGT-III	396	0,996	9168,597	1,228	2	gelding	17
16	OGT-IV	373	0,939	7967,091	1,067	2	gelding	17
16	OGT-V	391	0,984	6281,291	0,841	2	gelding	17
17	OGT-I	381	1,036	11010,177	0,564	2	gelding	17
17	OGT-II	390	1,061	24038,724	1,230	2	gelding	17
17	OGT-III	351	0,955	23298,711	1,192	2	gelding	17
17	OGT-IV	353	0,960	23463,636	1,201	2	gelding	17
17	OGT-V	363	0,987	15877,668	0,813	2	gelding	17

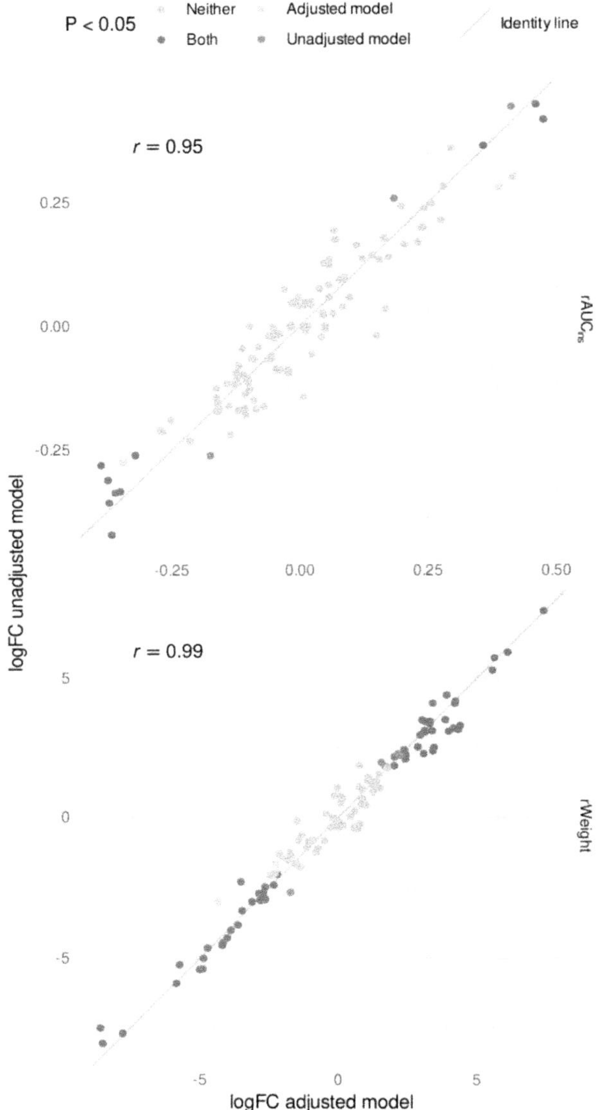

Figure S1 Scatterplot comparing the coefficients associated with rAUCins and rWeight in the adjusted and unadjusted linear models. The adjusted models include both predictors (rAUCins and rWeight), while the unadjusted models include only one them. The almost perfect agreement (high correlation along the identity line, $r \geq 0.95$) shows that the models are not affected by collinearity issues between rAUCins and rWeight.

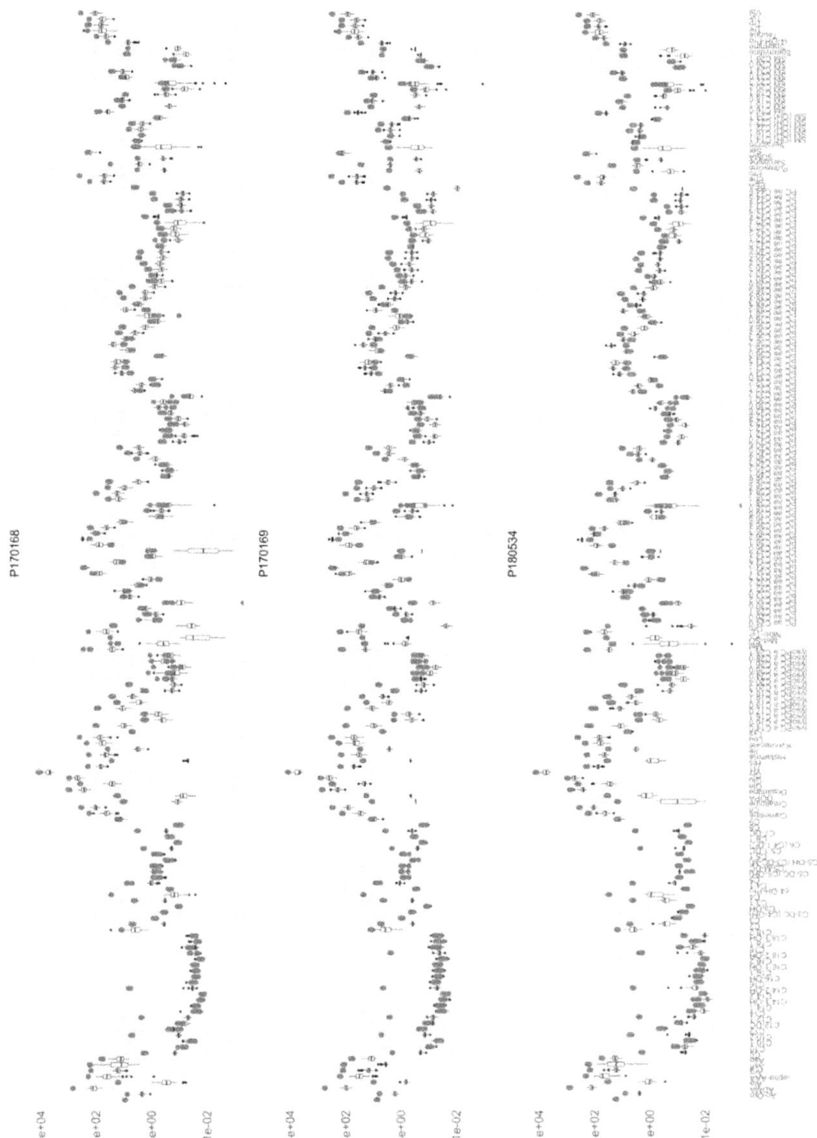

Figure S2 Comparison of the raw metabolite concentrations with the human QC samples. Boxplots of the raw sample data compared to the medium human QC (lyophilized human plasma with medium concentration levels). The plot is split in three parts (one for each measurement batch/assay plate). The boxplots contain all sample measurements for each metabolite and the human samples (which are technical replicates) are shown on top as red dots. Overall, the patterns are very close among batches and human levels are close to the equine ones a well.

5. Manuscript 4

Metabolic profile distinguishes laminitis-susceptible and -resistant ponies before and after feeding a high sugar diet

Julien Delarocque[1]*, Dania B. Reiche[2], Alexandra D. Meier[3], Tobias Warnken[1], Karsten Feige[1], Martin N. Sillence[3]

[1] Clinic for Horses, University of Veterinary Medicine Hannover, Foundation, Hannover, Germany.

[2] Boehringer Ingelheim Vetmedica, Ingelheim am Rhein, Germany.

[3] Biology and Environmental Science School, Queensland University of Technology, Queensland, Australia.

* Corresponding author

State of publication:

Published in BMC Veterinary Research (2021) 17:56
DOI: 10.1186/s12917-021-02763-7

Contributions to the manuscript:

Conceptualization: M.N.S., D.B.R., A.D.M; Methodology: J.D., D.B.R., M.N.S., T.W.; Formal analysis: J.D., D.B.R.; Investigation: A.D.M., M.N.S.; Resources: A.D.M., M.N.S, J.D., Data Curation: J.D., D.B.R., A.D.M.; Writing – original draft preparation: J.D., M.N.S., D.B.R.; Writing – review and editing: J.D., M.N.S., D.B.R., A.D.M., T.W., K.F.; Visualization: J.D.; Supervision: M.N.S., K.F.; Project administration: M.N.S.; Funding acquisition: M.N.S, D.B.R.

Delarocque *et al. BMC Veterinary Research* (2021) 17:56
https://doi.org/10.1186/s12917-021-02763-7

BMC Veterinary Research

RESEARCH ARTICLE

Open Access

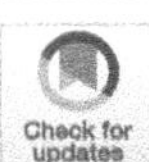

Metabolic profile distinguishes laminitis-susceptible and -resistant ponies before and after feeding a high sugar diet

Julien Delarocque[1*], Dania B. Reiche[2], Alexandra D. Meier[3], Tobias Warnken[1], Karsten Feige[1] and Martin N. Sillence[3]

Abstract

Background: Insulin dysregulation (ID) is a key risk factor for equine endocrinopathic laminitis, but in many cases ID can only be assessed accurately using dynamic tests. The identification of other biomarkers could provide an alternative or adjunct diagnostic method, to allow early intervention before laminitis develops. The present study characterised the metabolome of ponies with varying degrees of ID using basal and postprandial plasma samples obtained during a previous study, which examined the predictive power of blood insulin levels for the development of laminitis, in ponies fed a high-sugar diet. Samples from 10 pre-laminitic (PL – subsequently developed laminitis) and 10 non-laminitic (NL – did not develop laminitis) ponies were used in a targeted metabolomic assay. Differential concentration and pathway analysis were performed using linear models and global tests.

Results: Significant changes in the concentration of six glycerophospholipids (adj. $P \leq 0.024$) and a global enrichment of the glucose-alanine cycle (adj. $P = 0.048$) were found to characterise the response of PL ponies to the high-sugar diet. In contrast, the metabolites showed no significant association with the presence or absence of pituitary pars intermedia dysfunction in all ponies.

Conclusions: The present results suggest that ID and laminitis risk are associated with alterations in the glycerophospholipid and glucose metabolism, which may help understand and explain some molecular processes causing or resulting from these conditions. The prognostic value of the identified biomarkers for laminitis remains to be investigated in further metabolomic trials in horses and ponies.

Keywords: Laminitis, Equine metabolic syndrome, Pituitary pars intermedia dysfunction, Metabolome, Biomarker, Insulin dysregulation

Background

Insulin dysregulation (ID) is an endocrine disorder of horses and ponies, characterized by basal and/or postprandial hyperinsulinemia [1]. Prolonged hyperinsulinemia is associated with a high incidence of endocrinopathic laminitis (also known as insulin-associated laminitis), a painful and debilitating hoof condition, which in severe cases can necessitate euthanasia [2, 3]. While it is known that animals affected by ID may also suffer from equine metabolic syndrome (EMS) and/or pituitary *pars intermedia* dysfunction (PPID), the pathogenesis and detailed pathophysiology of ID are yet to be elucidated.

A relatively new approach to understanding complex disease processes is metabolomics [4]. This involves the

* Correspondence: julien.delarocque@tiho-hannover.de
[1]Clinic for Horses, University of Veterinary Medicine Hannover, Foundation, 30559 Hannover, Germany
Full list of author information is available at the end of the article

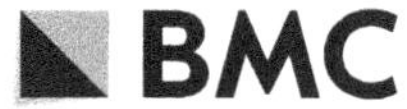

comprehensive analysis of disparate small molecules involved in cellular processes, and has already been used, for example, to identify metabolic pathways involved in disorders such as human metabolic syndrome or risk factors for the progression towards clinical diseases such as type 2 diabetes [5]. In recent years, metabolomic studies have increasingly been conducted in livestock as well [6]. The metabolic profile during an oral glucose test (OGT) has also been described in horses and ponies [7, 8].

Meanwhile, several models of insulin-associated laminitis have been developed [2, 3, 9, 10]. Among these, Meier et al. [10] described a method to induce laminitis in insulin-dysregulated ponies using a 'challenge diet' containing a high level of sugar and other non-structural carbohydrates (NSC). This method offers the advantage of exacerbating a pre-existing metabolic condition, using a natural dietary stimulus that resembles conditions that may be encountered in the field. The model corroborated the positive correlation between serum insulin concentrations and laminitis risk [10], and so several samples from that study were selected for further investigation using the metabolomics approach.

The present study used both basal plasma samples collected after an overnight fast a few days before the dietary challenge period, and postprandial samples collected 90 min after feeding the challenge diet, from ponies that subsequently did and did not develop laminitis. The primary aim of this retrospective study was to identify potential metabolic biomarkers, in addition to insulin, that may be associated with the onset or recurrence of laminitis. A second aim was to examine the effects of feeding in both groups, to determine if the power to predict laminitis was greater in samples from fed or fasted ponies, and/or to determine if feeding is a potential confounding factor. Finally, by identifying specific metabolites that differ in concentration according to laminitis risk, or which respond differently to feeding in both groups, we aimed to increase our understanding of the pathophysiology of ID.

Results

Data pre-processing

The 188 metabolites measured using the Biocrates AbsoluteIDQ p180 Kit belong to six substance classes. By summarising these classes and adding the kynurenine to tryptophan ratio (Kyn/Trp), 194 features were obtained. After pre-processing, 132 features were still present. Table 1 summarises the metabolites initially present and included in the analysis for each substance class. The number of samples varied between 10 and 20, depending on the hypothesis of interest. The characteristics of the sample population are described in an additional file (see Additional file 1). Fifteen missing values for threonine (Thr) had to be imputed using the *k*-nearest neighbours method.

Table 1 Summary of the metabolites present in the plasma of insulin-dysregulated ponies, grouped by chemical classes, before and after normalisation. Metabolites that were below the limit of detection in > 50% of samples, or which had a coefficient of variation within QC-samples > 20%, are excluded. Summary columns were added (i.e. sum of each class, except for sugars, and kynurenine:tryptophan ratio), resulting in 132 features included in the data analysis

Class	Before normalisation	After normalisation
Acylcarnitines	40	4
Amino acids	21	21
Biogenic amines	21	12
Glycerophospholipids	90	73
Sphingolipids	15	15
Sugars	1	1
Summary values	6	6
Total	194	132

From 188 metabolites, 181 could be associated with a metabolite identifier from the human metabolome database (HMDB) [11]. Of the 126 metabolites (without the summary values) included in the data analysis, 125 were associated with an HMDB identifier. Especially among lipids, one feature can correspond to several isomers because the assay relies on flow-injection analysis for some of the metabolite classes. In such cases the first best match from the HMDB database was used. Sixty-four HMDB identities could then be associated with 1006 unique metabolic pathways from the small molecule pathway database [12]. Twenty-one pathways, including at least three metabolites from the assay, were available for metabolite set enrichment analysis (MSEA).

Comparisons between pre-laminitic and non-laminitic ponies

Basal samples

Although principal component analysis (PCA) revealed a good separation between PL ($n = 5$) and NL ($n = 5$) ponies for basal samples (Fig. 1a), no significant differences were detected in individual metabolite concentrations (Additional file 2), indicating insufficient discriminatory power of single metabolites at group sizes of $n = 5$. Likewise, no significantly enriched pathways were identified.

Postprandial samples

Postprandial samples collected after feeding the high-NSC diet resulted in a moderate separation in PCA between PL ($n = 10$) and NL ($n = 10$) ponies (Fig. 1b), and the differential concentration of six glycerophospholipids (Fig. 2, Additional file 2). Additionally, the glucose-alanine cycle was found to be enriched (false discovery rate [FDR] adjusted $P = 0.048$), with hexoses (H1), glutamic acid (Glu) and alanine (Ala) being positively associated with eventual laminitis.

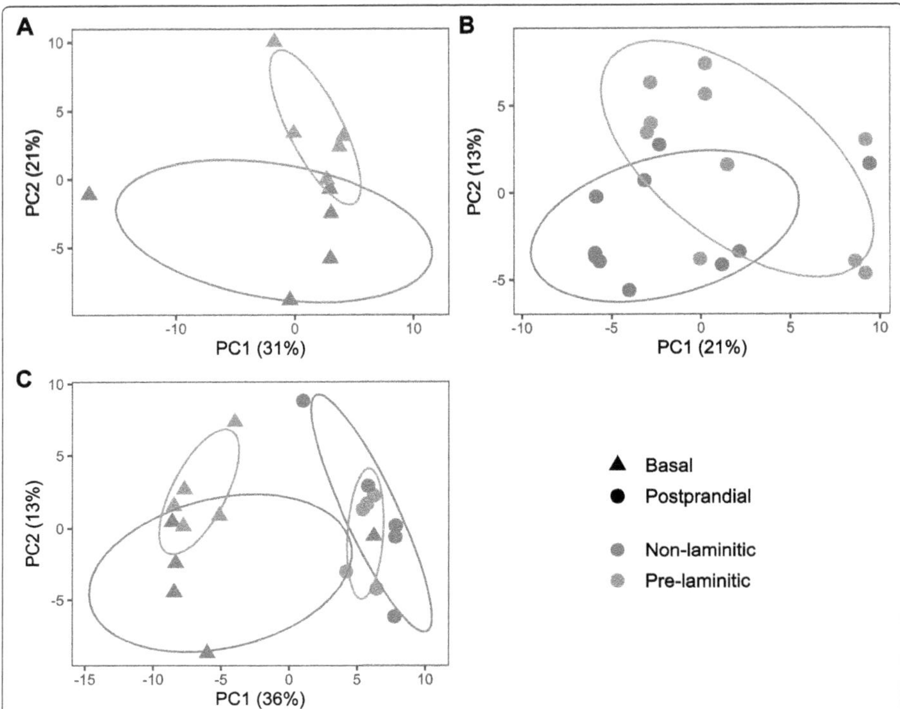

Fig. 1 Principal component analysis (PCA) of 132 metabolite concentrations in the plasma of ponies after an overnight fast (basal), or feeding a high-NSC diet (postprandial) from a cohort that contained a group of animals that subsequently developed laminitis (Pre-laminitic, red), and a group that did not (Non-laminitic, blue). To represent high dimensional data, PCA creates a linear combination of the dataset features such as to capture the maximum variance in the data. The amount of total variation explained by the two first principal components is given along the x and y axis, respectively. Each point represents one plasma sample from one pony either in the basal (triangle) or postprandial state (circle). The ellipses represent the 68% confidence interval of each group. The basal laminitic and non-laminitic samples (**a**) fell into two clusters which were best separated by features associated with PC2. In contrast, there was a greater overlap between the groups for the postprandial samples (**b**). When the factors of group and feeding were combined (**c**), some separation between groups was still evident for the basal samples, whereas the groups clustered together in the postprandial samples. A good separation between clusters indicates that it is possible to distinguish both groups by a linear combination of features

Interaction between feeding and propensity for laminitis

In PCA (Fig. 1c) the basal and postprandial samples separated well along the first principal component, indicating that feeding alone explains a significant amount of variation within the data. A separation between PL ($n = 5$) and NL ($n = 5$) ponies was visible in the basal samples, but not in the postprandial samples. Thus, it appears that feeding induces opposite shifts along the second principal component for each group, and has the potential to influence the interpretation of metabolomic data in regard to laminitis risk.

As indicated by analysis of differential concentration, four metabolites were associated with group differences in the response to feeding. Kynurenine and PC aa C30:2 increased in the NL group after feeding, but decreased in PL ponies; whereas PC aa C42:2 and PC ae C30:0 displayed the opposite pattern (Fig. 3, Additional file 2). These differences were not associated with any significantly enriched metabolic pathway.

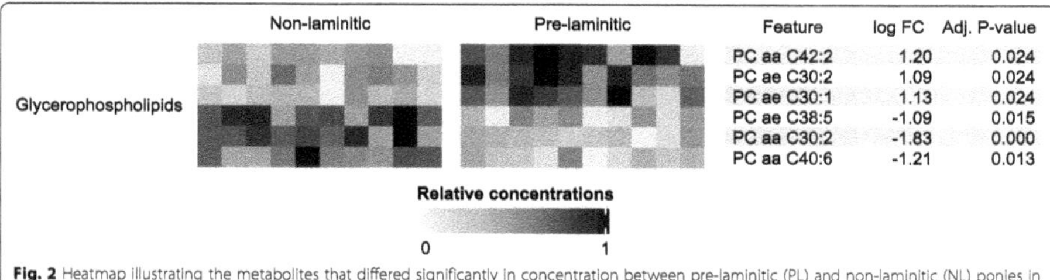

Fig. 2 Heatmap illustrating the metabolites that differed significantly in concentration between pre-laminitic (PL) and non-laminitic (NL) ponies in postprandial samples. Three phosphatidylcholines (PC) were positively associated with eventual laminitis (darker colours in the "Pre-laminitic" column and positive $\log_2$ fold change [log FC]) while three were negatively associated with this condition. A log FC of 1 indicates that the normalized metabolite concentration was twice as high in PL in comparison to NL ponies

Effect of PPID on the metabolic response to feeding

The separation of PPID ($n = 6$) and non-PPID ($n = 14$) ponies in PCA performed on the postprandial samples was weak to moderate, but also partly confounded by eventual laminitis (Additional file 3). No individual metabolites were affected significantly (Additional file 2) and no enriched pathways could be detected.

Association between insulin and the metabolome in postprandial samples

The association between insulin concentrations and the metabolic profile was investigated in several ways. In a full model, including the factors of group (NL and PL), insulin and a group x insulin interaction, the metabolic differences between groups were not significant. Insulin, however, showed a significant negative association with 6 amino acids and with the sum of amino acids. None of the metabolites revealed any significant group x insulin interaction. In contrast, when a subgroup analysis was performed, two more amino acids (valine and isoleucine; see Fig. 4 and Additional file 2 for the complete list) were significant in NL ponies ($n = 10$), while no metabolites were significant in PL ponies ($n = 10$). Driven by the strong negative association between insulin and several amino acids in NL ponies, 15 significantly enriched pathways could be detected (Table 2).

Discussion

The present study investigated metabolic differences in blood samples from a previous experiment [10], which included ponies with varying degrees of ID. One group of ponies in this cohort developed laminitis upon being fed a high-NSC diet, and a second group did not. Both basal and postprandial samples taken before the ponies eventually developed laminitis were analysed, to determine the effect of feeding alone, and to explore any feeding x group interactions.

Although PCA analysis revealed an obvious difference between the groups both before and after feeding, the number of basal samples was small, and the laminitis groups could not be differentiated on the basis of individual metabolites, or pathways, using the basal samples alone. When the larger number of postprandial samples was analysed, individual metabolites and certain

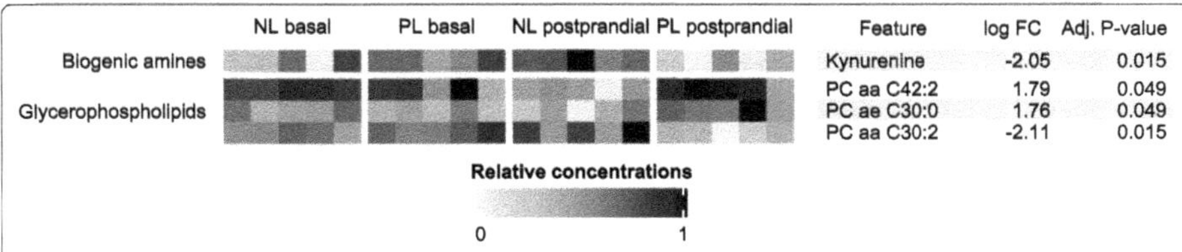

Fig. 3 Heatmap illustrating one biogenic amine and three glycerophospholipids that showed a significant association with subsequent laminitis in samples collected from ponies before and after feeding. Kynurenine concentrations were low in basal samples and increased postprandially in non-laminitic (NL) ponies, but showed the opposite pattern in ponies that subsequently developed laminitis (PL). Log FC is the $\log_2$ fold change of the difference of differences between basal and postprandial samples from both PL and NL groups. The features are grouped by functional classes. Two features decrease in PL while increasing in NL postprandially (kynurenine and PC aa C30:2), while the other two (positive logFC) show an opposite pattern

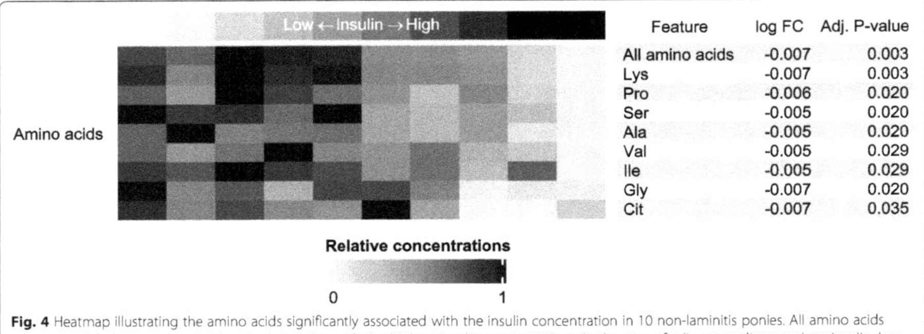

Fig. 4 Heatmap illustrating the amino acids significantly associated with the insulin concentration in 10 non-laminitis ponies. All amino acids were present in lower concentrations in the ponies with the highest insulin concentrations. In the case of a linear predictor such as insulin, log FC indicates the variation in units of normalized amino acid concentration for every unit of insulin (in μIU/mL), hence the small values

metabolic pathways were found to be associated with laminitis propensity. When investigating the feeding x group interaction, feeding alone had a marked effect on certain metabolites, masking the ability to differentiate between NL and PL ponies in postprandial samples using PCA alone. A considerable amount of variation in the data was explained by the variation in insulin concentrations. Unlike PL ponies, the postprandial metabolome of NL ponies displayed a negative association between amino acid and insulin concentrations. Lastly, no major impact on the metabolome due to the presence or absence of PPID could be detected.

Metabolites and pathways potentially associated with a propensity for laminitis

While no single metabolites or pathways that differentiate NL from PL ponies could be identified in basal samples in the present study, previous equine metabolomic studies have identified differences using basal samples, associated with hyperinsulinemia [7, 8], obesity and

Table 2 Metabolic pathways significantly enriched with increasing insulin concentrations. *P*-values are FDR adjusted. Metabolites included in each pathway are shown in bold when significantly contributing to the test result. The direction of association is indicated by (+) for a positive and (−) for a negative association with insulin. Despite being described as enrichment, variations in both directions are considered in absolute values, so that decreases in metabolite concentrations can result in significantly enriched pathways as well. Moreover, positive and negative associations within a pathway do not cancel each other out

Pathway	Adj. *P* value	Metabolites
Ammonia Recycling	0.001	**Ser** (−), **Gly** (−), **Asn** (−), **His** (−), Gln (−), Asp (−), Glu (+)
Glycine and Serine Metabolism	0.001	**Ser** (−), **Ala** (−), **Gly** (−), **Met** (−), Arg (−), Sarcosine (+), Glu (+)
Carnitine Synthesis	0.001	**Lys** (−), **Gly** (−), C0 (−)
Alanine Metabolism	0.002	**Ala** (−), **Gly** (−), Glu (+)
Urea Cycle	0.003	**Ala** (−), **Cit** (−), **Orn** (−), Arg (−), Gln (−), Asp (−), Glu (+)
Glutamate Metabolism	0.004	**Ala** (−), **Gly** (−), Gln (−), Asp (−), Glu (+)
Arginine and Proline Metabolism	0.004	**Pro** (−), **Gly** (−), **Cit** (−), **Orn** (−), Arg (−), Asp (−), Glu (+)
Valine, Leucine, and Isoleucine Degradation	0.009	**Val** (−), **Ile** (−), **Leu** (−), Glu (+)
Methionine Metabolism	0.011	**Ser** (−), **Gly** (−), **Met** (−), Met-SO (−), Putrescine (−), Sarcosine (+)
Glucose-Alanine Cycle	0.011	**Ala** (−), H1 (+), Glu (+)
Lysine Degradation	0.013	**Lys** (−), alpha-AAA (−), Glu (+)
Aspartate Metabolism	0.018	**Asn** (−), **Cit** (−), Arg (−), Gln (−), Asp (−), Glu (+)
Purine Metabolism	0.018	**Gly** (−), Gln (−), Asp (−), Glu (+)
beta-Alanine Metabolism	0.042	**His** (−), Carnosine (−), Asp (−), Glu (+)
Histidine Metabolism	0.045	**His** (−), Carnosine (−), Glu (+)

laminitis history [8]. However, the number of significant metabolites reported varied based on the statistical test used, or was not adjusted for multiple comparisons, so it remains unclear if the absence of significant results in the present case is due to a lack of power, a different set of analysed metabolites, or the absence of substantial basal metabolic impact of a propensity for laminitis. Nevertheless, the fact that there was a notable separation between both groups in PCA, indicates they may be differentiated by a linear combination of metabolite concentrations (i.e. using multivariate statistical methods such as discriminant analysis).

In postprandial samples, three phosphatidylcholines (PCs) were increased in PL ponies, while three others were decreased. While the glycerophospholipid profile (including phosphatidylcholines) is known to be affected by insulin and hepatic metabolism, it remains difficult to associate single molecules with specific pathways or pathomechanisms [13]. Moreover, the lipids reported in the present study could be indicators of disease as well as of an accurate response to a different stimulus (e.g. higher insulin levels). Nevertheless, PC ae C38:5 was decreased in PL and has previously been reported to be negatively associated with body mass index in humans [14]. While neither cresty neck score (CNS) or body condition score (BCS) were significantly higher in PL ponies (data not shown), this result could be explained by a higher body fat content, which might have been underestimated by BCS [15]. In contrast to the down-regulation of PC aa C42:2 described in cows with hepatic lipidosis [16], this metabolite was increased in PL ponies, which, as explained above, may also be an indicator of an hepatic insulin sensitivity. Likewise, observed enrichment of the glucose-alanine cycle could result from an increase in glucose resorption, or the inhibition of gluconeogenesis [17]. Interestingly, an increased gluconeogenesis from alanine and lactate, potentially relying on similar mechanisms, was observed in type 2 diabetes mellitus in humans [18].

In humans, PCs with a higher degree of unsaturation (higher number of double bounds) appear to protect from diabetes progression, whereas an increased risk is associated with higher contents of saturated fatty acid chains [19, 20]. Similar conclusions were reached by Ding and Rexrode [21] regarding the risk for cardiovascular diseases. Interestingly, such polyunsaturated PCs (PC ae C38:5, PC aa C40:6; Fig. 2) were higher in NL than PL ponies in postprandial samples in the present study.

Phosphatidylcholine PC aa C42:2 was present in similar concentrations in PL and NL ponies in the basal state, but decreased upon feeding the high NSC diet in NL ponies, while increasing in the PL ponies. In contrast, kynurenine, previously reported to increase following an OGT in horses [7], displayed the opposite pattern. Because an enzyme activated during inflammation (indoleamine 2,3-dioxygenase, IDO) catalyses one pathway of kynurenine synthesis from tryptophan [22], an increase in kynurenine can be associated with low-grade inflammation as reported during the OGT in horses [7], in lame cows [23], and in humans with metabolic syndrome [5]. However, since neither tryptophan nor the kynurenine:tryptophan ratio showed a significant variation, the present results are not indicative of inflammation in either group. Overall, it should be noted that the basal (pre-feeding) and postprandial samples were collected a few days apart, and it is possible this may have affected the results. Additionally, the postprandial samples included in this study are not necessarily directly comparable to samples taken during an OGT. Further, an impact of the high NSC diet on the microbiome, itself affecting the metabolome, cannot be excluded, even if samples were taken at the beginning of the dietary challenge. Indeed, the influence of the microbiome on markers of the glucose/insulin homeostasis has previously been described in horses [24, 25].

The comparison between postprandial and basal samples in the first two principal components of PCA indicated that group differences were more obvious in the basal state than postprandially, suggesting that feeding a high NSC diet lessens the metabolic differences. However, one should bear in mind that the metabolites included in the panel were selected to reflect energy metabolism and are not exhaustive of the equine metabolome. In contrast, although this could be attributable to a larger sample size, both groups were distinguished by more metabolites in postprandial samples in univariate analysis. As a result, it cannot be concluded that either postprandial or basal testing is more powerful to predict eventual laminitis based on the present results. Yet, since dynamic tests are preferred for the diagnosis of ID because they exacerbate its impact on insulin secretion [26], the relationship between insulin and the postprandial metabolome is of high interest.

Impact of insulin on the metabolome

A major and well described effect of insulin is the stimulation of amino acid uptake for protein synthesis, especially in muscle tissue [27]. During an OGT, amino acid concentrations in blood were shown to decrease in several species [7, 8, 28]; therefore the negative correlation between postprandial insulin and amino acid concentrations reported in the present study is expected. However, this effect was not detectable in PL ponies during subgroup analysis, suggesting some form of peripheral insulin resistance in this group. Since no group differences were found for amino acids when disregarding the insulin concentration, it is possible that this supposed insulin resistance was offset by hyperinsulinemia. To investigate this possibility further, the simultaneous assessment of ID and tissue-specific insulin sensitivity by immunoblotting [29], proteomics or hardly realisable (in horses) positron emission tomography in combination with a 18F fluorodeoxyglucose OGT [30] would be required.

The pathways associated with insulin are dominated by a restrained amino acid metabolism. Apart from glutamic acid (Glu), the results of this study further support enhanced protein synthesis. As blood insulin levels and BCS were slightly positively correlated ($\rho = 0.37$), it should be noted that Glu was positively associated with obesity in humans [31]. As a result, the (supposedly negative) effect of insulin on Glu may be offset by a positive effect of obesity.

Conclusions

Previous metabolomic studies around EMS and ID in ponies and horses have described the response to OGT depending upon insulinemia [7, 8], obesity, and history of laminitis [8]. To the authors' knowledge, however, this is the first study of the metabolome in relation to the future development of laminitis during a realistic dietary challenge. Six glycerophospholipids characterising the postprandial metabolome of PL ponies were identified as potential biomarkers for future risk of laminitis. Additionally, differences in the metabolic impact of insulin suggested that PL ponies have an insulin-sensitive hepatic metabolism, but insulin-resistant peripheral metabolism, which warrants further investigation on the proteomic level.

Due to the costs of such analyses, it was not possible to evaluate the predictive capabilities of these biomarkers (i.e. sensitivity and specificity) on additional samples in this study. Moreover, fewer samples were available for the differentiation of basal samples and to explore group x feeding interactions, negatively impacting the power of these analyses. Lastly, a genetic impact on the results cannot be excluded since only ponies were included in the present study. Further metabolomic investigations involving healthy, pre-laminitic and laminitic horses are warranted to clearly elucidate the prognostic value of these markers for laminitis in ponies with ID.

Methods

The samples used in this study were obtained from a previous prospective trial approved by the Animal Care and Ethics Committees of Queensland University of Technology (Brisbane, Australia, #1400000575) and The University of Queensland (St Lucia, Australia, #QUT/SVS/114/14), which investigated laminitis occurrence in ponies with ID fed a high-NSC diet. The ponies were purchased from local owners and dealers. At the end of the trial, the ponies were offered for adoption and successfully rehomed. The samples were selected from a larger set based on the phenotype and insulin response of the ponies to an oral glucose test [10]. To know the details of the experiment that gave rise to this work consult [10].

Animals

Due to cost constraints, subsets of samples were selected for metabolomic analysis to obtain balanced groups of eventually laminitic ($n = 10$) and non-laminitic ($n = 10$) ponies, based on their sex, dental age and diagnosis of PPID. At the time of sampling, none of the ponies had developed laminitis. Those who subsequently developed laminitis are classified here as PL; while those who remained sound are classed as NL. Basal samples were available in addition to the postprandial samples in five PL and five NL ponies, so that 30 samples were analysed in total. The characteristics of individual ponies in the sample population, including age, PPID status, season of sampling and insulin concentrations, are provided in an additional file (see Additional file 1).

Basal samples

The basal samples were obtained by jugular venipuncture at 8 AM, after overnight fasting, between 1 and 5 days before the start of the dietary challenge period. Blood (10 mL) was collected into both plain serum tubes (for the analysis of insulin) and into EDTA-coated tubes (for the analysis of adrenocorticotropic hormone (ACTH) and metabolomic analysis). Blood in the serum tubes was allowed to clot for 20 min at room temperature, before centrifugation. Plasma tubes were centrifuged immediately. All samples were stored in 1 ml aliquots at − 80 °C.

Postprandial samples

As described previously [10], during the dietary challenge period the ponies received a high-NSC diet of roasted-micronized oat flakes, lucerne (alfalfa) chaff, molasses and dextrose, which provided ~12 g/NSC/kg bodyweight/d. The feed was divided into three daily meals and was given for up to 18 days. Lucerne hay and a vitamin/mineral supplement were provided additionally, as a separate meal, so that the total ration included ~37% roughage. Postprandial samples were obtained on the morning of the second day of the challenge period, 90 min after feeding the first high-NSC meal. Blood was collected through a jugular catheter and processed as described above.

Insulin measurements
Serum samples were transported on the day of collection to QML Pathology (Brisbane, Queensland, Australia) for the analysis of insulin concentrations using an ADVIA Centaur chemiluminescent assay (Siemens Healthcare Diagnostics, Bayswater, Victoria, Australia) [32].

Diagnosis of PPID
The diagnosis or exclusion of PPID was based on a combination of clinical signs (hypertrichosis and polydipsia/polyuria) and basal ACTH concentrations using seasonally-adjusted cut-off values of > 27.8 pg/ml in non-autumn months and > 77.4 pg/ml in autumn months [33]. Adrenocorticotropic hormone levels were determined using the previously validated Immulite 2000 chemiluminescence method [34] by VetPath Laboratories (Ascot, Western Australia, Australia).

Laminitis detection
All ponies were examined daily during the dietary challenge period. At the first indication of pain or lameness, a laminitis examination was conducted and filmed. The recording was sent immediately to two blinded experts for scoring on a 12 point scale, using a modification of the Obel method developed by Meier et al. [35]. A diagnosis of laminitis was made when the average score was > 3. In such cases, the pony was immediately removed from the diet and provided with the best standard of care for laminitis treatment, as previously described [10].

Metabolomic assay
Metabolic profiling of the samples was performed at the Fraunhofer Institute of Toxicology and Experimental Medicine (ITEM, Hanover, Lower-Saxony, Germany) using a Biocrates AbsoluteIDQ p180 Kit (Biocrates Life Sciences AG, Innsbruck, Tyrol, Austria). This assay includes up to 188 metabolites related to glycolysis, oxidative processes, lipid degradation and inflammatory signalling. Amino acids and biogenic amines were measured by liquid chromatography (Agilent 1290 Infinity II LC, Santa Clara, CA, USA) tandem mass spectrometry (AB SCIEX 5500 QTrap mass spectrometer; AB SCIEX, Darmstadt, Germany), while acylcarnitines, hexoses, glycerophospholipids (PC and lysophosphatidylcholines), and sphingomyelins were quantified using flow injection analysis-tandem mass spectrometry.

Statistical analysis
Statistical analysis was performed using R 4.0.2 [36]. The metabolomic dataset was prepared by removing metabolites when more than 50% of the values were below the limit of detection (LOD). Remaining values below the LOD were set to half the value of the LOD. After aligning QC samples by "QC robust LOESS signal correction" [37], metabolites with a coefficient of variation within QC-samples greater than 20% were removed as well. Missing values were imputed by the *k*-nearest neighbours method [38]. After $\log_2$-transformation, the data were scaled (auto-scale) and quantile normalised [39].

Analysis of differential concentration was performed with the 'limma' R-package [40]. In essence, unpaired *t*-tests with pooled variance moderated by empirical Bayes were performed for each metabolite, to investigate (1) metabolic differences between PL and NL ponies in basal and postprandial samples, as well as the feeding x group interaction (represented by the difference between postprandial and basal samples), and (2) the impact of PPID on the postprandial metabolome. The association between insulin and the postprandial metabolome (3) was analysed using a moderated linear model for each subgroup.

Metabolite set enrichment analysis was conducted for each of the three hypotheses using the 'globaltest' package [41]. In global tests, the alternative hypothesis is that a set of covariates (in this case, the metabolites of a pathway) is globally associated with an outcome, in a way that many weak associations can become significant. This approach relies on logistic regression for binary outcomes (eventual laminitis or PPID) and linear regression for continuous outcomes (insulin).

Principal component analysis was performed for each of the hypotheses. All reported *P*-values were adjusted to control a FDR of 5% using the Benjamini-Hochberg procedure [42].

Supplementary Information
The online version contains supplementary material available at https://doi.org/10.1186/s12917-021-02763-7.

Additional file 1: Table S1. Characteristics of individual ponies in the sample population, including age, PPID status, season of sampling and insulin concentrations. Ten pre-laminitic (PL) and ten non-laminitic (NL) ponies were included in the study. Postprandial plasma samples were available from all ponies. Basal plasma samples were available for five NL and five PL ponies.

Additional file 2: Table S2. Top 10 metabolites from the linear models corresponding to each analysed hypothesis. The $\log_2$ fold change (logFC) is provided alongside its 95% confidence interval for each of the ten metabolites with lowest *p*-value. A positive logFC indicates higher metabolite concentrations in pre-laminitic or PPID ponies, or, for the feeding x group interaction, a stronger increase of metabolite concentrations in pre-laminitic ponies. *P*-values corresponding to a moderated *t*-statistic are given in addition to the FDR-adjusted *p*-value.

Additional file 3: Fig. S1. Principal component analysis from the postprandial samples. Ponies with PPID are shown in yellow; ponies without PPID are shown in green. The 68% confidence ellipse for each group is represented in the corresponding colour.

Abbreviations
ACTH: Adrenocorticotropic hormone; Ala: Alanine; alpha-AAA: Alpha-Aminoadipic acid; Arg: Arginine; Asn: Asparagine; Asp: Aspartate; BCS: Body condition score; C0: Carnitine; Cit: Citrulline; EMS: Equine metabolic

syndrome; FDR: False discovery rate; Gln: Glutamine; Glu: Glutamate; Gly: Glycine; H1: Sum of hexoses; His: Histidine; HMDB: Human metabolite database; ID: Insulin dysregulation; Ile: Isoleucine; Leu: Leucine; LOD: Limit of detection; Lys: Lysine; Met: Methionine; Met-SO: Methionine sulfoxide; MSEA: Metabolite set enrichment analysis; NL: Non-laminitic; NSC: Non-structural carbohydrate; OGT: Oral glucose test; Orn: Ornithine; PCA: Principal component analysis; PL: Pre-laminitic; PPID: Pituitary *pars intermedia* dysfunction; Pro: Proline; Ser: Serine; Val: Valine

Acknowledgements
Open Access funding enabled and organized by Projekt DEAL.

Authors' contributions
MNS, DBR and ADM designed the experiments. ADM and MNS performed the experiments. ADM, DBR, MNS, TW, KF and JD contributed to the acquisition of data. JD and DBR analysed the data. JD, DBR and MNS interpreted the results. JD, DBR and MNS drafted the manuscript. JD, DBR, ADM, TW, KF and MNS reviewed drafts of the paper. All authors read and accepted the final version of the manuscript.

Funding
This project was funded by Boehringer Ingelheim Vetmedica GmbH, Germany. Boehringer Ingelheim Vetmedica GmbH had a role in the study design and contributed to the preparation of the manuscript. This publication was supported by Deutsche Forschungsgemeinschaft and University of Veterinary Medicine Hannover, Foundation within the funding programme Open Access Publishing. No additional external funding was received.

Availability of data and materials
The dataset analysed during the current study is available from the corresponding author on reasonable request.

Ethics approval and consent to participate
The data presented here were obtained from blood samples collected during a study approved by the Animal Care and Ethics Committees of the University of Queensland (Approval # QUT/SVS/114/14) and Queensland University of Technology (Approval # 1400000575).

Consent for publication
Not applicable.

Competing interests
Dania Reiche is employed by Boehringer Ingelheim Vetmedica GmbH. All other authors have declared that no competing interests exist.

Author details
[1]Clinic for Horses, University of Veterinary Medicine Hannover, Foundation, 30559 Hannover, Germany. [2]Boehringer Ingelheim Vetmedica GmbH, 55216 Ingelheim am Rhein, Germany. [3]Biology and Environmental Science School, Queensland University of Technology, Brisbane, Queensland 4000, Australia.

Received: 14 September 2020 Accepted: 13 January 2021
Published online: 28 January 2021

References
1. Frank N, Tadros EM. Insulin dysregulation. Equine Vet J. 2014;46:103–12. https://doi.org/10.1111/evj.12169.
2. Asplin KE, Sillence MN, Pollitt CC, McGowan CM. Induction of laminitis by prolonged hyperinsulinaemia in clinically normal ponies. Vet J. 2007;174: 530–5. https://doi.org/10.1016/j.tvjl.2007.07.003.
3. de Laat M a, CM MG, Sillence MN, Pollitt CC. Equine laminitis: induced by 48 h hyperinsulinaemia in Standardbred horses. Equine Vet J. 2010;42:129–35. https://doi.org/10.2746/042516409X475779.
4. Wishart DS. Metabolomics for investigating physiological and pathophysiological processes. Physiol Rev. 2019;99:1819–75. https://doi.org/10.1152/physrev.00035.2018.
5. Lent-Schochet D, McLaughlin M, Ramakrishnan N, Jialal I. Exploratory metabolomics of metabolic syndrome: a status report. World J Diabetes. 2019;10:23–36. https://doi.org/10.4239/wjd.v10.i1.23.
6. Goldansaz SA, Guo AC, Sajed T, Steele MA, Plastow GS, Wishart DS. Livestock metabolomics and the livestock metabolome: a systematic review. PLoS One. 2017;12:1–26. https://doi.org/10.1371/journal.pone.0177675.
7. Kenéz WT, Feige K, Huber K. Lower plasma trans-4-hydroxyproline and methionine sulfoxide levels are associated with insulin dysregulation in horses. BMC Vet Res. 2018. https://doi.org/10.1186/s12917-018-1479-z.
8. Jacob SI, Murray KJ, Rendahl AK, Geor RJ, Schultz NE, McCue ME. Metabolic perturbations in welsh ponies with insulin dysregulation, obesity, and laminitis. J Vet Intern Med. 2018;32:1215–33. https://doi.org/10.1111/jvim.15095.
9. Garner HE, Moore JN, Johnson JH, Clark L, Amend JF, Tritschler LG, et al. Changes in the Caecal Flora associated with the onset of laminitis. Equine Vet J. 1978;10:249–52. https://doi.org/10.1111/j.2042-3306.1978.tb02273.x.
10. Meier AD, de Laat MA, Reiche DB, Pollitt CC, Walsh DM, McGree JM, et al. The oral glucose test predicts laminitis risk in ponies fed a diet high in nonstructural carbohydrates. Domest Anim Endocrinol. 2018;63:1–9. https://doi.org/10.1016/j.domaniend.2017.10.008.
11. Wishart DS, Feunang YD, Marcu A, Guo AC, Liang K, Vázquez-Fresno R, et al. HMDB 4.0: the human metabolome database for 2018. Nucleic Acids Res. 2018;46:D608–17. https://doi.org/10.1093/nar/gkx1089.
12. Jewison T, Su Y, Disfany FM, Liang Y, Knox C, Maclejewski A, et al. SMPDB 2.0: big improvements to the small molecule pathway database. Nucleic Acids Res. 2014;42:478–84. https://doi.org/10.1093/nar/gkt1067.
13. Chang W, Hatch GM, Wang Y, Yu F, Wang M. The relationship between phospholipids and insulin resistance: from clinical to experimental studies. J Cell Mol Med. 2019;23:702–10. https://doi.org/10.1111/jcmm.13984.
14. Wallace M, Morris C, O'Grada CM, Ryan M, Dillon ET, Coleman E, et al. Relationship between the lipidome, inflammatory markers and insulin resistance. Mol BioSyst. 2014;10:1586–95. https://doi.org/10.1039/C3MB70529C.
15. Dugdale AH, Grove-White D, Curtis GC, Harris PA, Argo CM. Body condition scoring as a predictor of body fat in horses and ponies. Vet J. 2012;194:173–8. https://doi.org/10.1016/j.tvjl.2012.03.024.
16. Imhasly S, Naegeli H, Baumann S, von Bergen M, Luch A, Jungnickel H, et al. Metabolomic biomarkers correlating with hepatic lipidosis in dairy cows. BMC Vet Res. 2014;10. https://doi.org/10.1186/1746-6148-10-122.
17. Felig P. The glucose-alanine cycle. Metabolism. 1973;22:179–207. https://doi.org/10.1016/0026-0495(73)90269-2.
18. Consoli A, Nurjhan N, Reilly JJ, Bier DM, Gerich JE. Mechanism of increased gluconeogenesis in noninsulin-dependent diabetes mellitus. Role of alterations in systemic, hepatic, and muscle lactate and alanine metabolism. J Clin Invest. 1990;86:2038–45. https://doi.org/10.1172/JCI114940.
19. Rhee EP, Cheng S, Larson MG, Walford GA, Lewis GD, McCabe E, et al. Lipid profiling identifies a triacylglycerol signature of insulin resistance and improves diabetes prediction in humans. J Clin Invest. 2011;121:1402–11. https://doi.org/10.1172/JCI44442.
20. Floegel A, Stefan N, Yu Z, Mühlenbruch K, Drogan D, Joost HG, et al. Identification of serum metabolites associated with risk of type 2 diabetes using a targeted metabolomic approach. Diabetes. 2013;62:639–48. https://doi.org/10.2337/db12-0495.
21. Ding M, Rexrode KM. A review of lipidomics of cardiovascular disease highlights the importance of isolating lipoproteins. Metabolites. 2020;10:1–13. https://doi.org/10.3390/metabo10040163.
22. Mangge H, Summers KL, Meinitzer A, Zelzer S, Almer G, Prassl R, et al. Obesity-related dysregulation of the tryptophan-Kynurenine metabolism: role of age and parameters of the metabolic syndrome. Obesity. 2014;22: 195–201. https://doi.org/10.1002/oby.20491.
23. Zhang G, Zwierzchowski G, Mandal R, Wishart DS, Ametaj BN. Serum metabolomics identifies metabolite panels that differentiate lame dairy cows from healthy ones. Metabolomics. 2020;16:1–22. https://doi.org/10.1007/s11306-020-01693-z.
24. Biddle AS, Tomb JF, Fan Z. Microbiome and blood analyte differences point to community and metabolic signatures in lean and obese horses. Front Vet Sci. 2018;5:12–4. https://doi.org/10.3389/fvets.2018.00225.
25. Coleman MC, Whitfield-Cargile CM, Madrigal RG, Cohen ND. Comparison of the microbiome, metabolome, and lipidome of obese and non-obese horses. PLoS One. 2019;14:1–17. https://doi.org/10.1371/journal.pone.0215918.
26. Durham AE, Frank N, McGowan CM, Menzies-Gow NJ, Roelfsema E, Vervuert I, et al. ECEIM consensus statement on equine metabolic syndrome. J Vet Intern Med. 2019;33:335–49. https://doi.org/10.1111/jvim.15423.
27. Kimball SR, Farrell PA, Jefferson LS. Invited review: role of insulin in translational control of protein synthesis in skeletal muscle by amino acids

or exercise. J Appl Physiol. 2002;93:1168–80. https://doi.org/10.1152/japplphysiol.00221.2002.

28. Ho JE, Larson MG, Vasan RS, Ghorbani A, Cheng S, Rhee EP, et al. Metabolite profiles during oral glucose challenge. Diabetes. 2013;62:2689–98. https://doi.org/10.2337/db12-0754.
29. Warnken T, Brehm R, Feige K, Huber K. Insulin signaling in various equine tissues under basal conditions and acute stimulation by intravenously injected insulin. Domest Anim Endocrinol. 2017;61:17–26. https://doi.org/10.1016/j.domaniend.2017.04.003.
30. Johansson E, Lubberink M, Heurling K, Eriksson JW, Skrtic S, Ahlström H, et al. Whole-body imaging of tissue-specific insulin sensitivity and body composition by using an integrated PET/MR system: a feasibility study. Radiology. 2018;286:271–8. https://doi.org/10.1148/radiol.2017162949.
31. Bagheri M, Farzadfar F, Qi L, Yekaninejad MS, Chamari M, Zeleznik OA, et al. Obesity-related Metabolomic profiles and discrimination of metabolically unhealthy obesity. J Proteome Res. 2018;17:1452–62. https://doi.org/10.1021/acs.jproteome.7b00802.
32. Warnken T, Huber K, Feige K. Comparison of three different methods for the quantification of equine insulin. BMC Vet Res. 2016;12:196. https://doi.org/10.1186/s12917-016-0828-z.
33. McGowan TW, Pinchbeck GP, McGowan CM. Prevalence, risk factors and clinical signs predictive for equine pituitary pars intermedia dysfunction in aged horses. Equine Vet J. 2013;45:74–9. https://doi.org/10.1111/j.2042-3306.2012.00578.x.
34. Köller G, Bassewitz K, Schusser GF. Referenzbereiche von Insulin, insulinähnlichem Wachstumsfaktor 1 (IGF-1) und adrenokortikotropem Hormon bei Ponys. Tierarztl Prax Ausgabe G Grosstiere - Nutztiere. 2016;44:19–25. https://doi.org/10.15653/TPG-150428.
35. Meier A, de Laat M, Pollitt C, Walsh D, McGree J, Reiche DB, et al. A "modified Obel" method for the severity scoring of (endocrinopathic) equine laminitis. PeerJ. 2019;7:e7084. https://doi.org/10.7717/peerj.7084.
36. R Core Team. R: A Language and Environment for Statistical Computing 2020.
37. Dunn WB, Broadhurst D, Begley P, Zelena E, Francis-Mcintyre S, Anderson N, et al. Procedures for large-scale metabolic profiling of serum and plasma using gas chromatography and liquid chromatography coupled to mass spectrometry. Nat Protoc. 2011;6:1060–83. https://doi.org/10.1038/nprot.2011.335.
38. Hastie T, Tibshirani R, Sherlock G, Eisen M, Brown P, Botstein D. Imputing missing data for gene expression arrays; 1999.
39. Bolstad BM, Irizarry R, Astrand M, Speed TP. A comparison of normalization methods for high density oligonucleotide array data based on variance and bias. Bioinformatics. 2003;19:185–93. https://doi.org/10.1093/bioinformatics/19.2.185.
40. Ritchie ME, Phipson B, Wu D, Hu Y, Law CW, Shi W, et al. Limma powers differential expression analyses for RNA-sequencing and microarray studies. Nucleic Acids Res. 2015;43:e47. https://doi.org/10.1093/nar/gkv007.
41. Goeman JJ, van de Geer SA, van Houwelingen HC. Testing against a high dimensional alternative. J R Stat Soc Ser B Stat Methodol. 2006;68:477–93. https://doi.org/10.1111/j.1467-9868.2006.00551.x.
42. Benjamini Y, Hochberg Y. Controlling the false discovery rate: a practical and powerful approach to multiple testing. J R Stat Soc Ser B. 1995;57:289–300. https://doi.org/10.2307/2346101.

Publisher's Note

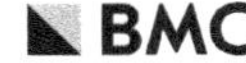

Additional files

Table S1 Characteristics of individual ponies in the sample population, including age, PPID status and insulin concentrations. Ten pre-laminitic (PL) and ten non-laminitic (NL) ponies were included in the study. Postprandial plasma samples were available from all ponies. Basal plasma samples were available for five NL and five PL ponies.

Pony ID	Group	Sex	PPID	Dental age (yrs)	Height (cm)	Season of sampling	Basal insulin (µIU/ml)	Postprandial insulin (µIU/ml)
034	PL	Mare	no	13	115	Spring	6	369
087	PL	Gelding	yes	16	93	Autumn	5	319
027	PL	Gelding	yes	15	114	Autumn	10	222
043	PL	Gelding	yes	22	102	Summer	8	205
023	PL	Mare	no	13	83	Winter	11	198
091	PL	Mare	no	10	82	Summer		583
002	PL	Gelding	yes	16	132	Winter		360
116	PL	Gelding	yes	20	122	Autumn		250
009	PL	Mare	no	20	123	Winter		180
003	PL	Gelding	no	10	102	Winter		160
030	NL	Mare	no	10	122	Spring	7	169
042	NL	Gelding	no	10	124	Autumn	6	76
133	NL	Gelding	no	7	81	Autumn	4	62
033	NL	Gelding	no	22	145	Spring	1	62
102	NL	Mare	yes	20	81	Autumn	4	47
124	NL	Gelding	no	18	102	Autumn		440
071	NL	Mare	no	15	142	Autumn		366
029	NL	Gelding	no	16	145	Spring		268
064	NL	Mare	no	11	125	Autumn		195
127	NL	Mare	no	10	91	Autumn		81

Table S2 Top 10 metabolites from the linear models corresponding to each analysed hypothesis. The log_2 fold change (logFC) is provided alongside its 95% confidence interval for each of the ten metabolites with lowest p-value. A positive logFC indicates higher metabolite concentrations in pre-laminitic or PPID ponies, or, for the feeding x group interaction, a stronger increase of metabolite concentrations in pre-laminitic ponies. P-values corresponding to a moderated t-statistic are given in addition to the FDR-adjusted p-value.

Metabolite	Class	HMDB ID	logFC	CI.low	CI.upp	t	P value	adj.P val
Basal top 10								
lysoPC a C18:1	glycerophospholipids	HMDB0002815	1,482	0,587	2,377	3,399	0,002	0,149
lysoPC a C16:0	glycerophospholipids	HMDB0010382	1,547	0,607	2,487	3,378	0,002	0,149
lysoPC a C18:0	glycerophospholipids	HMDB0010384	1,461	0,519	2,402	3,184	0,004	0,150
PC aa C30:0	glycerophospholipids	HMDB0011203	-1,270	-2,113	-0,426	-3,090	0,005	0,150
lysoPC a C18:2	glycerophospholipids	HMDB0010386	1,171	0,323	2,020	2,834	0,009	0,150
Leu	amino acids	HMDB0000687	1,274	0,351	2,198	2,833	0,009	0,150
lysoPC a C16:1	glycerophospholipids	HMDB0010383	1,180	0,315	2,044	2,802	0,009	0,150
SM C18:0	sphingolipids	HMDB0012087	-1,263	-2,196	-0,330	-2,779	0,010	0,150
biogenic amines	biogenic amines		-1,173	-2,044	-0,302	-2,763	0,010	0,150
lysoPC a C17:0	glycerophospholipids	HMDB0012108	1,141	0,228	2,054	2,565	0,016	0,201

Metabolite	Class	HMDB ID	logFC	CI.low	CI.upp	t	P value	adj.P val
Post-prandial top 10								
PC aa C30:2	glycerophospholipids	HMDB0007999	-1,829	-2,459	-1,200	-5,943	0,000	0,000
PC aa C40:6	glycerophospholipids	HMDB0008121	-1,206	-1,787	-0,625	-4,244	0,000	0,013
PC ae C38:5	glycerophospholipids	HMDB0013432	-1,086	-1,632	-0,540	-4,063	0,000	0,015
PC ae C30:2	glycerophospholipids	HMDB0013410	1,091	0,492	1,690	3,725	0,001	0,024
PC aa C42:2	glycerophospholipids	HMDB0008092	1,200	0,525	1,875	3,635	0,001	0,024
PC ae C30:1	glycerophospholipids	HMDB0013402	1,134	0,494	1,774	3,623	0,001	0,024
PC ae C30:0	glycerophospholipids	HMDB0013341	1,122	0,361	1,882	3,013	0,005	0,088
PC aa C38:6	glycerophospholipids	HMDB0008147	-0,957	-1,607	-0,307	-3,009	0,005	0,088
SM C22:3	sphingolipids	HMDB0013468	-0,820	-1,399	-0,241	-2,894	0,007	0,104
PC aa C38:1	glycerophospholipids	HMDB0008269	-0,864	-1,495	-0,233	-2,798	0,009	0,119
Feeding x Group interaction top 10								
PC aa C30:2	glycerophospholipids	HMDB0007999	-2,114	-3,151	-1,078	-4,077	0,000	0,015
Kynurenine	biogenic amines	HMDB0000684	-2,050	-3,097	-1,003	-3,914	0,000	0,015
PC ae C30:0	glycerophospholipids	HMDB0013341	1,757	0,701	2,812	3,327	0,001	0,049
PC aa C42:2	glycerophospholipids	HMDB0008092	1,793	0,715	2,872	3,324	0,001	0,049
Kyn/Trp			-1,658	-2,729	-0,587	-3,095	0,003	0,078
Gly	amino acids	HMDB0000123	-1,611	-2,706	-0,516	-2,941	0,005	0,101
Thr	amino acids	HMDB0000167	-1,445	-2,524	-0,366	-2,678	0,009	0,171
lysoPC a C18:1	glycerophospholipids	HMDB0002815	-1,361	-2,411	-0,312	-2,593	0,012	0,171
amino acids	amino acids		-1,367	-2,428	-0,305	-2,574	0,012	0,171
PC aa C30:0	glycerophospholipids	HMDB0011203	1,323	0,276	2,370	2,526	0,014	0,171
Insulin top 10								
All amino acids	amino acids		-0,007	-0,009	-0,004	-6,018	0,000	0,003
Lys	amino acids	HMDB0000182	-0,007	-0,010	-0,004	-5,693	0,000	0,003
Ser	amino acids	HMDB0000187	-0,005	-0,008	-0,003	-4,308	0,001	0,020
Ala	amino acids	HMDB0000161	-0,005	-0,008	-0,003	-4,219	0,001	0,020
Gly	amino acids	HMDB0000123	-0,007	-0,010	-0,003	-4,190	0,001	0,020
Pro	amino acids	HMDB0000162	-0,006	-0,008	-0,003	-4,094	0,001	0,020
Ile	amino acids	HMDB0000172	-0,005	-0,009	-0,002	-3,778	0,002	0,029
Val	amino acids	HMDB0000883	-0,005	-0,007	-0,002	-3,772	0,002	0,029
Cit	amino acids	HMDB0000904	-0,007	-0,011	-0,003	-3,623	0,002	0,035
PC ae C34:3	glycerophospholipids	HMDB0013413	0,003	0,001	0,006	3,190	0,006	0,078
PPID top 10								
PC aa C30:2	glycerophospholipids	HMDB0007999	-1,124	-2,059	-0,188	-2,457	0,020	0,668
PC aa C34:4	glycerophospholipids	HMDB0007884	-0,695	-1,299	-0,091	-2,353	0,026	0,668
sphingolipids	sphingolipids		-0,795	-1,505	-0,085	-2,289	0,030	0,668
Orn	amino acids	HMDB0000214	1,053	0,108	1,997	2,279	0,030	0,668
Sarcosine	biogenic amines	HMDB0000271	1,079	0,090	2,067	2,232	0,033	0,668
PC ae C36:2	glycerophospholipids	HMDB0013418	-0,642	-1,239	-0,046	-2,202	0,036	0,668
PC ae C32:1	glycerophospholipids	HMDB0013404	-0,749	-1,466	-0,032	-2,137	0,041	0,668
lysoPC a C18:0	glycerophospholipids	HMDB0010384	0,605	0,013	1,197	2,090	0,046	0,668
H1	sugars	HMDB0000122	0,686	-0,001	1,373	2,043	0,050	0,668
Gln	amino acids	HMDB0000641	0,697	-0,002	1,396	2,039	0,051	0,668

Figure S1 Principal component analysis from the post-prandial samples. Ponies with PPID are shown in yellow; ponies without PPID are shown in green. The 68% confidence ellipse for each group is represented in the corresponding colour.

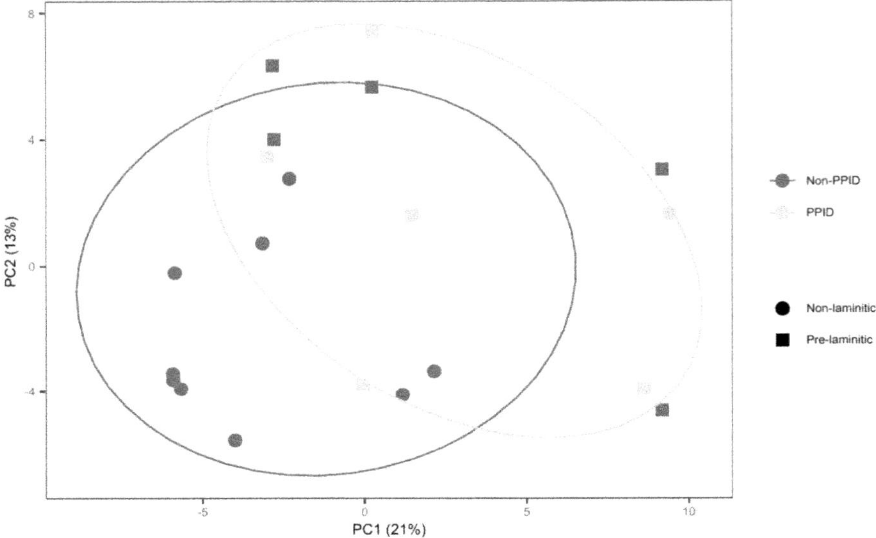

6. General discussion

After describing the metabolic impact of ID and the OGT, the relationship between variations in bodyweight, the level of ID and the metabolome was characterised. Additionally, associations between the metabolic profile and subsequent development of laminitis during a high-sugar dietary challenge were uncovered. The objectives of this discussion will be to synthesize the main conclusions of these manuscripts into the following points:

(1) to summarize which candidate biomarkers for ID and laminitis were identified in the different manuscripts and their potential diagnostic use,

(2) to describe what conclusions could be drawn from the use of the OGT as a model of HI,

(3) to compare the metabolic impact of weight gain and of fluctuations in ID,

(4) to list potential pathomechanisms associated with ID corroborated by its metabolic profile, and

(5) to suggest future directions for the investigation of the pathomechanisms of ID.

6.1. Potential biomarkers of insulin dysregulation and laminitis

In the first manuscript, the total insulin response to the OGT was approximated by the area under the curve of insulin, AUC_{ins}, as surrogate to ID. Potential biomarkers correlated with the insulin response were identified using two statistical approaches. The phosphatidylcholine (PC) PC ae C38:6, arginine (Arg), carnitine (C0), acetylcarnitine (C2), the sum of acylcarnitines and spermidine were linearly associated with the insulin response (Figure 1, manuscript 1). Additional candidate biomarkers were found by partial least-squares discriminant analysis (PLS-DA), when the horses were split in two groups ('low' and 'high') based on their insulin response (Figure 2, manuscript 1). Acetylcarnitine and the sum of acylcarnitines were identified using both methods. It is difficult to compare these results to the other manuscripts, as almost no acylcarnitines met the requirements of quality control in the subsequent metabolomic measurements (**Figure 2**). However, the negative association between carnitine and the total insulin response contrasts with the higher carnitine concentrations reported in ponies with ID by Jacob *et al.* (although not necessarily significant, since the estimates were not adjusted for multiple comparisons) [85].

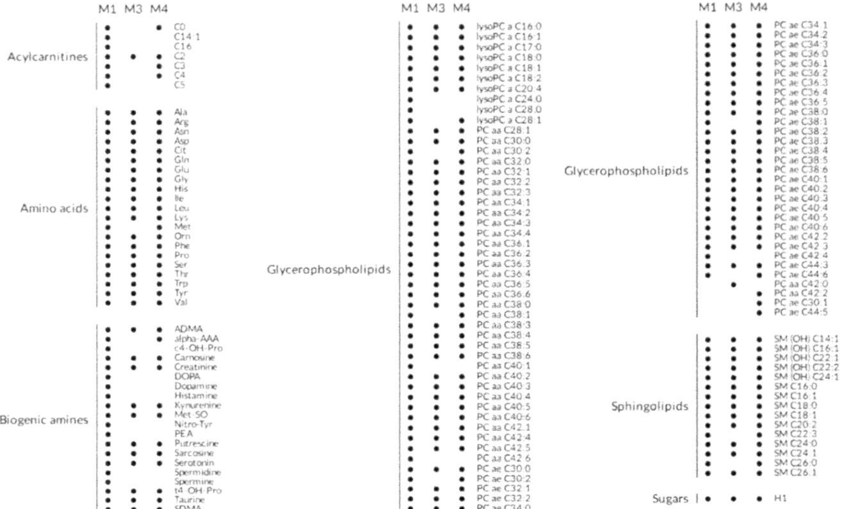

Figure 2 Comparison of the metabolites available for statistical analysis in each of the manuscripts. The metabolites a grouped by biochemical classes. The inclusion of the metabolites in the manuscripts is represented by a bullet (•) in the corresponding column (M1 for manuscript 1 and so forth). The same assay, covering 188 metabolites, was used for each manuscript. Since some metabolites were excluded during the quality-control process, their results are not always comparable. Only metabolites represented in at least one of the manuscripts are shown. Manuscript 1 was the most comprehensive, with 139 metabolites (excluding summary values).

The predictive potential of these biomarkers was evaluated in a proof-of-concept approach based on the bootstrap using baseline samples only (Figure 3, manuscript 1). The aim was to select a few metabolites which may later be brought to a diagnostic panel for ID requiring only a basal blood sample. Since the OGT and other similar protocols are laborious and time-consuming, such panel would ideally provide an adjunct or alternative diagnostic method, while being economically more accessible than a full metabolomic assay. Best model performance was obtained for 7 and 20 metabolites. Nevertheless, such an approach would first require validating the present results using the targeted platform (e.g., a point of care device) in an independent cohort.

In the fourth manuscript, the clinical relevance was increased by putting the focus on subsequent laminitis rather than ID. Several phosphatidylcholines were highlighted as candidate biomarkers in the postprandial samples. In contrast, no baseline differences could be identified by univariate methods. On the other hand, the clusters observed in the principal component analysis (PCA) of the baseline samples corresponded to the outcome of subsequent laminitis, indicating that it may be possible to distinguish both groups by a linear combination of some of the metabolite concentrations. With sample sizes of n = 5 or n = 10, some of the questions addressed in this manuscript might suffer from a lack of statistical power, rather than from the absence of a biological effect. It is difficult to compare the results associated with ID and with subsequent laminitis because most of the respective metabolites of interest were not represented in both manuscripts.

6.2. The oral glucose test as hyperinsulinemia model

The OGT-protocol used during the experiments included in this thesis relied on the administration of 0.5 g/kg glucose *via* nasogastric intubation and succeeded in inducing HI in horses. Fitzgerald *et al.* reported that the insulin concentrations after two hours on pasture correlated well with the insulin response to an in-feed OGT protocol with 0.75 g/kg glucose, while slightly overestimating it [9]. The lower glucose dosage used in the present study might alleviate this bias.

The metabolic impact of the OGT itself is relevant to assess the safety of the protocol – as one would not want to induce laminitis during the test – but could also provide insights on the events occurring during natural HI. In manuscript 1, the factor directly associated with glucose influx and insulin secretion is 'Time'. Indeed, the area under the curve of insulin (AUC_{ins}) comprises the full insulin response and is therefore an indicator of ID rather than of the dynamics of the OGT. Accordingly, the AUC_{ins} associated with the basal, 120, and 180 min samples of a horse during an OGT is constant.

The metabolites significantly associated with the pharmacokinetics and dynamics of glucose intake and insulin secretion are presented in Figure 1A of manuscript 1. Overall, the metabolic profile during the OGT corresponds to the expectations, with an opposite time-course of carnitine (C0) and acetylcarnitine (C2), which can be attributed to a decrease in β-oxidation upon glucose influx and a decrease of amino acid concentrations upon insulin secretion, as described during the OGT in humans [114]. However, the tryptophan:kynurenine ratio was found to increase over time, possibly indicating an activation of the indoleamine 2,3-dioxygenase (IDO), which is considered to indicate low-grade inflammation and was also associated with the human metabolic syndrome [82,115]. These results corroborate a previous report of increasing kynurenine concentrations during the OGT in horses [84]. While such variations were not reported in manuscript 4, it should be noted that the basal (pre-feeding) and postprandial samples were collected a few days apart, which might have induced additional variation. Provided that the OGT accurately models natural HI, these results could support the hypothesis of inflammation during HI. Each hyperinsulinemic episode could damage the lamellar epithelium and/or prime its metabolism for further decisive events in the onset of laminitis.

Lastly, the increase of dihydroxyphenylalanin (DOPA, a precursor of dopamine) during the OGT generated the hypothesis that a possible lack of inhibition of the insulin secretion in the β-cells of the pancreatic islets by DOPA and dopamine [116,117] could link PPID and ID. Indeed, Parkinson's disease is associated with a loss of dopaminergic innervation in several brain areas which is similar to the loss of dopaminergic inhibition in the pars intermedia of the pituitary gland of horses with PPID [118], and incidentally, Parkinson's disease is also associated with glucose intolerance and type 2 diabetes mellitus [119,120]. As DOPA was not among the metabolites conforming to the quality-control requirements in the subsequent trials, the results cannot be compared with regard to this point.

The OGT as a model of HI is only partly comparable to the alimentary model of laminitis induction used in the fourth manuscript. First, the purpose of these models differs, secondly, a comparison between both models was not a primary aim of the study so that there are methodological differences, and lastly, the sets of metabolites available for statistical analysis differed. Interestingly, the metabolite PC aa C40:6 was relevant to both the identification of horses with a high insulin response (Figure 2, manuscript 1) and to the distinction between laminitis-prone and resistant ponies in postprandial samples (Figure 2, manuscript 4). Increased PC aa C40:6 concentrations were previously associated with coronary artery disease in humans [121], as opposed to the decrease associated with ID and susceptibility to laminitis in the present work. Assuming that this metabolite is related to endothelial metabolism, this finding could be linked to vascular dysfunction, which was previously shown to be associated with ID [52,122] and suspected to be involved in the pathogenesis of laminitis. The opposite changes associated with ID and coronary artery disease might be explained by the distinct pathomechanism. Nevertheless, such hypotheses remain clearly speculative.

6.3. Insulin dysregulation in the context of the equine metabolic syndrome

As mentioned previously, EMS is a collection of risk factors for endocrinopathic laminitis, among which obesity plays a prominent role. While weight loss and weight gain were shown to have an opposite impact on ID or IR numerous times [15,57,98,101,123–128], these reports did not describe the nature of the relationship between body weight and insulin response to its full extent. Manuscript 2 was able to establish that weight variations have a proportional impact on the insulin response (Figure 2, manuscript 2). This relationship remained true in already normally conditioned, non-hyperinsulinemic horses. This suggests that there is no threshold above which the metabolism changes. It could be speculated that the proportion of metabolically active tissue (e.g., relative muscle and fat mass) plays a role here, although this parameter was not assessed during the trial. Additionally, the variance in the estimated effect of weight loss reported in multiple studies on this subject demonstrates that it is difficult to generalise the findings obtained using a specific protocol. Indeed, besides methodological aspects, any of the previously discussed factors affecting EMS might have influenced the results reported in these studies.

After having shown that the relationship between weight lost and reduction of the insulin response to OGT was linear, these data were coupled to metabolomics analyses in an attempt to disentangle the respective impact of weight gain and worsening of ID on the metabolome. To compare the first and third manuscript, it is essential to bear in mind the difference between AUC_{ins}, used as a surrogate to the level of ID in the first manuscript, and $rAUC_{ins}$, which describes the variation in the level of ID as compared to the mean level of ID in the third manuscript. Most interestingly, some metabolites previously associated with ID, showed a stronger association with weight gain (an increase of rWeight) than with $rAUC_{ins}$.

One such metabolite is arginine (Figure 1, manuscript 1; Figure 1, manuscript 3), which is essentially known as potent insulin secretagogue [129] and precursor of nitric oxide (NO) [130]. In contrast to the negative association between AUC_{ins} and arginine reported in the first manuscript, a positive correlation with $rAUC_{ins}$ was observed in the third manuscript but was exceeded by the negative correlation with rWeight. Having shown that a variation of rWeight is associated with the five-fold variation in $rAUC_{ins}$ in the second manuscript, the fold changes associated with both factors can be compared. Even after applying this multiplicative factor, the absolute impact of rWeight on arginine outweighs the impact of $rAUC_{ins}$ on arginine. This explains why when bodyweight is not accounted for in the model, parts of the effect of bodyweight appears to be associated with the insulin response, as it was the case in the first manuscript. While weight gain usually is accompanied by a worsening of ID, it has been shown that there is a lean phenotype of EMS [56] and that obesity is not *per se* a cause of IR [57]. Studying these phenotypes could help further extricate the respective impact of weight gain and worsening of ID on the metabolic phenotype.

The ability of arginine to stimulate insulin production [129] might explain its positive association with $rAUC_{ins}$. Decreased arginine levels were previously associated with diabetes in humans [131] and obesity appears to increase asymmetric dimethylarginine, leading to a relative arginine deficiency [132]. However, hyperinsulinemia also reduces ADMA levels [133], which was corroborated in the first manuscript (Figure 2, manuscript 1), so that it is difficult to translate these findings to horses.

The molecule trans-4-hydroxyproline (t4-OH-Pro) was negatively associated with body mass index (BMI) in humans [134] and with ID in horses (where the impact of obesity was not analysed) [84]. Since obesity is a major risk factor for ID, these results appear compatible with the decrease of hydroxyproline associated with weight gain in manuscript 3.

The metabolome, the bodyweight and the level of ID are interrelated in complex ways, which might obfuscate previously assumed relationships. The objective of the present section was to describe how the simultaneous analysis of several factors can help distinguish their respective impact on the metabolome. Nevertheless, interventional studies targeting single metabolites are more suitable to establish causal relationships than metabolomic approaches.

6.4. Pathological processes potentially associated with insulin dysregulation

Several metabolites have been emphasized as potential biomarkers for ID or weight gain throughout this thesis. While it is currently not possible to establish if these metabolic abnormalities are a cause or a consequence of the associated conditions, potential pathomechanisms will be extrapolated from the information available on similar metabolic disorders in this section.

Hydroxyproline is obtained by posttranslational proline hydroxylation (mostly within collagen), which requires the antioxidant ascorbic acid [135]. It has therefore been hypothesized, that hydroxyproline is an indirect marker of oxidative stress [84]. However, the molecule also appears to exhibit direct inhibition of free radicals [136,137]. In manuscript 3, this metabolite was negatively associated with weight gain.

Arginine is a precursor of NO, which is a potent vasodilator and essential to vascular function [130]. In manuscript 1, arginine and its metabolites putrescine and spermidine were negatively associated with the total insulin response. It was shown in manuscript 3, that this apparent association might rather result from the effect of weight gain. Nonetheless, these observations could corroborate the previously reported vascular dysfunction associated with ID [52].

Lower carnitine levels were reported in obese humans with higher plasma fatty acid concentrations and attributed to increased carnitine dissipation through β-oxidation [138,139]. Carnitine facilitated weight loss [140] and improved insulin sensitivity [141] in humans, although the effects in horses were equivocal [142,143]. Nevertheless, the results presented in the first manuscript suggest that carnitine does play a role in ID.

Less is known about the metabolism of PCs as compared to the previously mentioned metabolites. There is some evidence that PCs with a higher degree of unsaturation (higher number of double bounds) appear to offer protection against a progression towards diabetes [144,145] or regarding the risk for cardiovascular diseases [146]. Interestingly, such polyunsaturated PCs (PC ae C38:5, PC aa C40:6; Figure 2, manuscript 4) were higher in laminitis-resistant than laminitis-prone ponies in postprandial samples. However, PC ae C38:6 was also positively associated with the total insulin response in the first manuscript (Figure 1, manuscript 1).

While the metabolites associated with subsequent laminitis in postprandial samples (Figure 2, manuscript 4) could not be associated with a specific pathway, a concurrent enrichment of the glucose-alanine cycle could be observed. This result could indicate an increase in glucose resorption, or the inhibition of gluconeogenesis [147]. An increased gluconeogenesis from alanine and lactate, compatible with the present findings, was observed in type 2 diabetes mellitus in humans [148], suggesting that the laminitis-prone ponies relied on additional pathways of gluconeogenesis as compared to the laminitis-resistant ones. Additionally, the correlations between insulin and the metabolome were less strong in laminitis-prone ponies as compared to laminitis-resistant ones, which is compatible with IR.

The kynurenine:tryptophan ratio and DOPA were associated with the response to the OGT independently of ID. As described earlier, the kynurenine-pathway is partly activated during inflammation [82,115]. In the present context, it could mean that the OGT induces low-grade inflammation, which could also be present during naturally occurring HI. The dopamine-precursor DOPA is on the other hand known to modulate the pancreatic insulin secretion [116]. The observed reduction in DOPA could result from regulatory mechanisms inhibiting the DOPA and dopamine associated insulin-depression secondary to glucose-influx. To the author's knowledge, this is the first time that DOPA is described in connection with the insulin response in horses and suggest a role for this pathway of insulin-modulation. Since horses with PPID suffer from a lack of dopaminergic inhibition of the pituitary *pars intermedia* [118], one could imagine that the inhibition of insulin secretion by DOPA is blunted in horses with PPID.

6.5. Future perspectives

Metabolomics approaches are bound to generate many hypotheses which require further exploration. For example, the use of biomarkers within point-of-care devices in the context of ID and laminitis would require validating the present findings on the targeted platform before being able to estimate biomarker performance on an independent cohort. In this respect, the first 20 metabolites identified by the baseline PLS-DA model appear promising.

The confirmation of the hypothesized molecular pathomechanisms associated with ID could be performed using various approaches. As an example, the β-cell response to arginine, dopamine and DOPA could be determined on isolated pancreatic islets from healthy and insulin-dysregulated horses. Further, the arginine metabolism could be described using methods of protein analysis on liver and kidney biopsies and correlated with the level of insulin dysregulation. More broadly, the transcriptome of various organs could be assessed under glucose and/or insulin stimulation.

The OGT as a model of HI has proven valuable in identifying biomarkers of ID. However, a better characterisation of this model might help in the interpretation of the results. For example, the enteral component of ID activated during the OGT could be assessed by comparing the metabolic response to intravenous glucose to oral glucose intake. In order to assess the validity of this model regarding pasture-associated laminitis, it could also be of interest to compare the metabolic response to grazing and the metabolic response to the OGT. The dynamics of glucose and grass intake are obviously different and it can be expected that the microbiome will react in another way to grass than to glucose.

Lastly, the role of carnitine and arginine has been emphasized several times throughout the thesis. These molecules are available as dietary supplements which could be used in horses. One could expect carnitine supplementation to affect the lipid and energy metabolism, while the impact of arginine on its metabolite and/or vascular function could be assessed.

7. Conclusion

The present thesis allowed to derive candidate biomarkers for ID. Additionally, potentially pathological mechanisms induced during the OGT or by HI (H1) were uncovered. Having shown that weight loss leads to a proportional reduction of the level of ID (H2), the independent impact of these two parameters on the metabolome was pointed out (H3). Lastly, several metabolites predicting subsequent laminitis were identified (H4), although the involved mechanisms (H5) are rather indicative of peripheral IR than novel pathways of laminitis.

The obtained results were analysed using more complex statistical methods than in earlier reports on the subject, such as mixed linear models and metabolite set enrichment analysis. As a result, the previously established effect of weight loss on ID could be shown to be proportional. The use of the OGT as a model to induce HI allowed to distinguish the immediate response to insulin from the differential response associated with ID (insulin *versus* total insulin response, AUC_{ins}).

Several new hypotheses regarding the pathophysiology of ID were formulated. Besides uncovering the prominent role of arginine and its metabolites, it was hypothesized that DOPA plays a role in the modulation of the insulin response in horses, which could link PPID and ID. Additionally, the previously reported activation of IDO during the OGT was further supported. The thereby corroborated induction of low-grade inflammation remains to be confirmed in naturally occurring HI. Finally, the use of candidate biomarkers was assessed in a proof-of-concept approach.

The knowledge on ID and EMS is currently essentially limited to phenotypic aspects while few is known about their pathomechanisms. Therefore, metabolic profiling is an interesting tool to describe metabolic consequences of these conditions. On the other hand, it is limited in helping to determine the molecular mechanisms at work when used alone. Therefore, methods from the fields of proteomics, transcriptomics, and genomics could be used additionally.

8. References

[1] Karikoski NP, Patterson-Kane JC, Asplin KE, McGowan TW, McNutt M, Singer ER, et al. Morphological and cellular changes in secondary epidermal laminae of horses with insulin-induced laminitis. Am J Vet Res 2014;75:161–8.

[2] Heymering HW. A Historical Perspective of Laminitis. Vet Clin North Am Equine Pract 2010;26:1–11.

[3] Obel N. Studies on the histopathology of acute laminitis. 1948.

[4] Jeffcott LB, Field JR, McLean JG, O'Dea K. Glucose tolerance and insulin sensitivity in ponies and Standardbred horses. Equine Vet J 1986;18:97–101.

[5] Frank N, Tadros EM. Insulin dysregulation. Equine Vet J 2014;46:103–12.

[6] Karikoski NP, Horn I, McGowan TW, McGowan CM. The prevalence of endocrinopathic laminitis among horses presented for laminitis at a first-opinion/referral equine hospital. Domest Anim Endocrinol 2011;41:111–7.

[7] Johnson PJ, Wiedmeyer CE, LaCarrubba A, Ganjam VK, Messer NT th. Diabetes, insulin resistance, and metabolic syndrome in horses. J Diabetes Sci Technol 2012;6:534–40.

[8] Johnson PJ, Wiedmeyer CE, Messer NT, Ganjam VK. Medical implications of obesity in horses--lessons for human obesity. J Diabetes Sci Technol 2009;3:163–74.

[9] Fitzgerald DM, Walsh DM, Sillence MN, Pollitt CC, de Laat MA. Insulin and incretin responses to grazing in insulin-dysregulated and healthy ponies. J Vet Intern Med 2018;33:225–32.

[10] de Laat MA, McGree JM, Sillence MN. Equine hyperinsulinemia: investigation of the enteroinsular axis during insulin dysregulation. Am J Physiol - Endocrinol Metab 2015;310:ajpendo.00362.2015.

[11] Borer KE, Bailey SR, Menzies-Gow NJ, Harris PA, Elliott J. Effect of feeding glucose, fructose, and inulin on blood glucose and insulin concentrations in normal ponies and those predisposed to laminitis. J Anim Sci 2012;90:3003–13.

[12] Bertin FR, de Laat MA. The diagnosis of equine insulin dysregulation. Equine Vet J 2017;49:570–6.

[13] Warnken T, Delarocque J, Schumacher S, Huber K, Feige K. Retrospective analysis of insulin responses to standard dosed oral glucose tests (OGTs) via naso-gastric tubing towards definition of an objective cut-off value. Acta Vet Scand 2018;60:4.

[14] Argo CMCG, Curtis GC, Grove-White D, Dugdale AHA, Barfoot CF, Harris PA. Weight loss resistance: A further consideration for the nutritional management of obese Equidae. Vet J 2012;194:179–88.

[15] Van Weyenberg S, Hesta M, Buyse J, Janssens GPJ. The effect of weight loss by energy restriction on metabolic profile and glucose tolerance in ponies. J Anim Physiol Anim Nutr (Berl) 2008;92:538–45.

[16] Delarocque J, Frers F, Huber K, Feige K, Warnken T. Weight loss is linearly associated with a reduction of the insulin response to an oral glucose test in Icelandic horses. BMC Vet Res 2020;16:151.

[17] Hoffman RM, Kronfeld DS, Cooper WL, Harris PA. Glucose clearance in grazing mares is affected by diet, pregnancy, and lactation. J Anim Sci 2003;81:1764–71.

[18] Smith S, Harris PA, Menzies-Gow NJ. Comparison of the in-feed glucose test and the oral sugar test. Equine Vet J 2016;48:224–7.

[19] Lindåse S, Nostell K, Askerfelt I, Bröjer J. A modified oral sugar test for evaluation of insulin and glucose dynamics in horses. Acta Vet Scand Anim Obes - Causes, Consequences Comp Asp Meet Abstr 2015;57:O4.

[20] Warnken T, Huber K, Feige K. Comparison of three different methods for the quantification of equine insulin. BMC Vet Res 2016;12:196.

[21] Banse HE, McCann J, Yang F, Wagg C, McFarlane D. Comparison of two methods for measurement of equine insulin. J Vet Diagn Invest 2014;26:527–30.

[22] Öberg J, Bröjer J, Wattle O, Lilliehöök I. Evaluation of an equine-optimized enzyme-linked immunosorbent assay for serum insulin measurement and stability study of equine serum insulin. Comp Clin Path 2011;21:1291–300.

[23] Borer-Weir KE, Bailey SR, Menzies-Gow NJ, Harris PA, Elliott J. Evaluation of a commercially available radioimmunoassay and species-specific ELISAs for measurement of high concentrations of insulin in equine serum. Am J Vet Res 2012;73:1596–602.

[24] Carslake HB, Pinchbeck GL, McGowan CM. Evaluation of a Chemiluminescent Immunoassay for Measurement of Equine Insulin. J Vet Intern Med 2017;31:568–74.

[25] Tinworth KD, Wynn PC, Boston RC, Harris PA, Sillence MN, Thevis M, et al. Evaluation of commercially available assays for the measurement of equine insulin. Domest Anim Endocrinol 2011;41:81–90.

[26] Johnson PJ. The equine metabolic syndrome peripheral Cushing's syndrome. Vet Clin North Am Equine Pr 2002;18:271–93.

[27] Frank N, Geor RJJ, Bailey SRR, Durham AEE, Johnson PJJ, American College of Veterinary Internal M. Equine metabolic syndrome. J Vet Intern Med 2010;24:467–75.

[28] Durham AE, Frank N, McGowan CM, Menzies-Gow NJ, Roelfsema E, Vervuert I, et al. ECEIM consensus statement on equine metabolic syndrome. J Vet Intern Med 2019;33:335–49.

[29] McFarlane D. Equine pituitary pars intermedia dysfunction. Vet Clin North Am Equine Pr 2011;27:93–113.

[30] Morgan RA, Keen JA, Homer N, Nixon M, McKinnon-Garvin AM, Moses-Williams JA, et al. Dysregulation of Cortisol Metabolism in Equine Pituitary Pars Intermedia Dysfunction. Endocrinology 2018;159:3791–800.

[31] Morgan RA, McGowan TW, Mcgowan CM. Prevalence and risk factors for hyperinsulinaemia in ponies in Queensland, Australia. Aust Vet J 2014;92:101–6.

[32] Muno JD. Prevalence, risk factors and seasonality of plasma insulin concentrations in normal horses in central Ohio. The Ohio State University, 2009.

[33] Pleasant RSS, Suagee JKK, Thatcher CDD, Elvinger F, Geor RJJ. Adiposity, plasma insulin, leptin, lipids, and oxidative stress in mature light breed horses. J Vet Intern Med 2013;27:576–82.

[34] Giles SL, Rands SA, Nicol CJ, Harris PA. Obesity prevalence and associated risk factors in outdoor living domestic horses and ponies. PeerJ 2014;2:e299.

[35] Thatcher CD, Pleasant RS, Geor RJ, Elvinger F, Negrin KA, Franklin J, et al. Prevalence of obesity in mature horses: an equine body condition study. J Anim Physiol Anim Nutr 2008;92:222.

[36] Ireland JL, McGowan CM. Epidemiology of pituitary pars intermedia dysfunction: A systematic literature review of clinical presentation, disease prevalence and risk factors. Vet J 2018;235:22–33.

[37] Wylie CE, Collins SN, Verheyen KLP, Richard Newton J. Frequency of equine laminitis: A systematic review with quality appraisal of published evidence. Vet J 2011;189:248–56.

[38] Asplin KE, Sillence MN, Pollitt CC, McGowan CM. Induction of laminitis by prolonged hyperinsulinaemia in clinically normal ponies. Vet J 2007;174:530–5.

[39] de Laat M a, McGowan CM, Sillence MN, Pollitt CC. Equine laminitis: induced by 48 h hyperinsulinaemia in Standardbred horses. Equine Vet J 2010;42:129–35.

[40] De Laat MA, Sillence MN, McGowan CM, Pollitt CC. Continuous intravenous infusion of glucose induces endogenous hyperinsulinaemia and lamellar histopathology in Standardbred horses. Vet J 2012;191:317–22.

[41] Carter RA, Treiber KH, Geor RJ, Douglass L, Harris PA. Prediction of incipient pasture-associated laminitis from hyperinsulinaemia, hyperleptinaemia and generalised and localised obesity in a cohort of ponies. Equine Vet J 2009;41:171–8.

[42] Treiber K, Carter R, Gay L, Williams C, Geor R. Inflammatory and redox status of ponies with a history of pasture-associated laminitis. Vet Immunol Immunopathol 2009;129:216–20.

[43] Meier AD, de Laat MA, Reiche DB, Pollitt CC, Walsh DM, McGree JM, et al. The oral glucose test predicts laminitis risk in ponies fed a diet high in nonstructural carbohydrates. Domest Anim Endocrinol 2018;63:1–9.

[44] Walsh DM, McGowan CM, McGowan T, Lamb S V., Schanbacher BJ, Place NJ. Correlation of Plasma Insulin Concentration with Laminitis Score in a Field Study of Equine Cushing's Disease and Equine Metabolic Syndrome. J Equine Vet Sci 2009;29:87–94.

[45] Karikoski NP, Mcgowan CM, Singer ER, Asplin KE, Tulamo R-M, Patterson-Kane JC. Pathology of Natural Cases of Equine Endocrinopathic Laminitis Associated With Hyperinsulinemia. Vet Pathol 2014;52:945–56.

[46] Menzies-Gow NJ, Harris PA, Elliott J. Prospective cohort study evaluating risk factors for the development of pasture-associated laminitis in the United Kingdom. Equine Vet J 2017;49:300–6.

[47] Kaur J. A comprehensive review on metabolic syndrome. Cardiol Res Pract 2014;2014.

[48] Shanik MH, Xu Y, Skrha J, Dankner R, Zick Y, Roth J. Insulin resistance and hyperinsulinemia: is hyperinsulinemia the cart or the horse? Diabetes Care 2008;31 Suppl 2.

[49] de Laat MA, Kyaw-Tanner MT, Sillence MN, McGowan CM, Pollitt CC. Advanced glycation endproducts in horses with insulin-induced laminitis. Vet Immunol Immunopathol 2012;145:395–401.

[50] Asplin KE, Curlewis JD, McGowan CM, Pollitt CC, Sillence MN. Glucose transport in the equine hoof. Equine Vet J 2011;43:196–201.

[51] Venugopal CS, Eades S, Holmes EP, Beadle RE. Insulin resistance in equine digital vessel rings: An in vitro model to study vascular dysfunction in equine laminitis. Equine Vet J 2011;43:744–9.

[52] Morgan RA, Keen JA, Walker BR, Hadoke PWF. Vascular dysfunction in horses with endocrinopathic laminitis. PLoS One 2016;11:1–14.

[53] Lane HE, Burns TA, Hegedus OC, Watts MR, Weber PS, Woltman KA, et al. Lamellar events related to insulin-like growth factor-1 receptor signalling in two models relevant to endocrinopathic laminitis. Equine Vet J 2017;49:643–54.

[54] Kullmann A, Weber PS, Bishop JB, Roux TM, Norby B, Burns TA, et al. Equine insulin receptor and insulin-like growth factor-1 receptor expression in digital lamellar tissue and insulin target tissues. Equine Vet J 2016;48:626–32.

[55] Jacob SI, Geor RJ, Weber PSD, Harris PA, McCue ME. Effect of age and dietary carbohydrate profiles on glucose and insulin dynamics in horses. Equine Vet J 2017;38:42–9.

[56] Bailey SR, Habershon-Butcher JL, Ransom KJ, Elliott J, Menzies-Gow NJ. Hypertension and insulin resistance in a mixed-breed population of ponies predisposed to laminitis. Am J Vet Res 2008;69:122–9.

[57] Bamford NJ, Potter SJ, Harris PA, Bailey SR. Effect of increased adiposity on insulin sensitivity and adipokine concentrations in horses and ponies fed a high fat diet, with or without a once daily high glycaemic meal. Equine Vet J 2016;48:368–73.

[58] Frank N, Elliott SB, Brandt LE, Keisler DH. Physical characteristics, blood hormone concentrations, and plasma lipid concentrations in obese horses with insulin resistance. J Am Vet Med Assoc 2006;228:1383–90.

[59] Coleman MC, Walzem RL, Kieffer AJ, Minamoto T, Suchodolski J, Cohen ND. Novel lipoprotein density profiling in laminitic, obese, and healthy horses. Domest Anim Endocrinol 2019;68:92–9.

[60] Auyyuenyong R, Henze A, Ungru J, Schweigert FJ, Raila J, Vervuert I. Determination of lipid profiles in serum of obese ponies before and after weight reduction by using multi-one-dimensional thin-layer chromatography. Res Vet Sci 2018;117:111–7.

[61] McCue ME, Geor RJ, Schultz N. Equine metabolic syndrome: A complex disease influenced by genetics and the environment. J Equine Vet Sci 2015;35:367–75.

[62] Cartmill JA. Leptin in Horses: Influences of Body Condition, Gender, Insulin Insensitivity, Feeding, and Dexamethasone. Louisiana State University, 2004.

[63] Wooldridge AA, Edwards HG, Plaisance EP, Applegate R, Taylor DR, Taintor J, et al. Evaluation of high-molecular weight adiponectin in horses. Am J Vet Res 2012;73:1230–40.

[64] Meier AD, de Laat MA, Reiche DB, Sillence MN. Glucagon-like peptide-1, insulin-like growth factor-1, and adiponectin in insulin-dysregulated ponies: effects of feeding a high nonstructural carbohydrate diet and association with prospective laminitis. Domest Anim Endocrinol 2019:106397.

[65] Fitzgerald DM, Anderson ST, Sillence MN, De Laat MA. The cresty neck score is an independent predictor of insulin dysregulation in ponies. PLoS One 2019;14:1–15.

[66] Kearns CF, McKeever KH, Roegner V, Brady SM, Malinowski K. Adiponectin and leptin are related to fat mass in horses. Vet J 2006;172:460–5.

[67] Geor RJ. Current concepts on the pathophysiology of pasture-associated laminitis. Vet Clin North Am Equine Pr 2010;26:265–76.

[68] Vick MM, Adams AA, Murphy BA, Sessions DR, Horohov DW, Cook RF, et al. Relationships among inflammatory cytokines, obesity, and insulin sensitivity in the horse. J Anim Sci 2007;85:1144–55.

[69] Wray H, Elliott J, Bailey SR, Harris PA, Menzies-Gow NJ. Plasma concentrations of inflammatory markers in previously laminitic ponies. Equine Vet J 2013;45:546–51.

[70] Tadros EM, Frank N, Donnell RL. Effects of equine metabolic syndrome on inflammatory responses of horses to intravenous lipopolysaccharide infusion. Am J Vet Res 2013;74:1010–9.

[71] Valle E, Storace D, Sanguineti R, Carter R, Odetti P, Geor R, et al. Association of the glycoxidative stress marker pentosidine with equine laminitis. Vet J 2013;196:445–50.

[72] Banse HE, Schultz N, McCue M, Geor R, McFarlane D. Comparison of two methods for measurement of equine adrenocorticotropin. J Vet Diagnostic Investig 2018;30:233–7.

[73] Campolo A, de Laat MA, Keith L, Gruntmeir KJ, Lacombe VA. Prolonged hyperinsulinemia affects metabolic signal transduction markers in a tissue specific manner. Domest Anim Endocrinol 2016;55:41–5.

[74] Warnken T, Brehm R, Feige K, Huber K. Insulin signaling in various equine tissues under basal conditions and acute stimulation by intravenously injected insulin. Domest Anim Endocrinol 2017;61:17–26.

[75] de Laat MA, Clement CK, Sillence MN, McGowan CM, Pollitt CC, Lacombe VA. The impact of prolonged hyperinsulinaemia on glucose transport in equine skeletal muscle and digital lamellae. Equine Vet J 2015;47:494–501.

[76] Timpson AJ, de Mestre AM, Elliott J, Harris PA, Cheng Z, Mirczuk SM, et al. Seasonal and Dietary Influences on Adipose Tissue and Systemic Gene Expression in Control and Previously Laminitic Ponies. J Equine Vet Sci 2018;69:84–95.

[77] Burns TA, Watts MR, Weber PS, McCutcheon LJ, Geor RJ, Belknap JK. Laminar inflammatory events in lean and obese ponies subjected to high carbohydrate feeding: Implications for pasture-associated laminitis. Equine Vet J 2015;47:489–93.

[78] Elzinga S, Wood P, Adams AA. Plasma Lipidomic and Inflammatory Cytokine Profiles of Horses With Equine Metabolic Syndrome. J Equine Vet Sci 2016;40:49–55.

[79] Siard-Altman MH, Harris PA, Moffett-Krotky AD, Ireland JL, Betancourt A, Barker VD, et al. Relationships of inflamm-aging with circulating nutrient levels, body composition, age, and pituitary pars intermedia dysfunction in a senior horse population. Vet Immunol Immunopathol 2020;221:110013.

[80] Kheder MH, Bailey SR, Dudley KJ, Sillence MN, de Laat MA. Equine glucagon-like peptide-1 receptor physiology. PeerJ 2018;6:e4316.

[81] Ungru J, Blüher M, Coenen M, Raila J, Boston R, Vervuert I. Effects of body weight reduction on blood adipokines and subcutaneous adipose tissue adipokine mRNA expression profiles in obese

ponies. Vet Rec 2012;171:528.

[82] Lent-Schochet D, McLaughlin M, Ramakrishnan N, Jialal I. Exploratory metabolomics of metabolic syndrome: A status report. World J Diabetes 2019;10:23–36.

[83] Goldansaz SA, Guo AC, Sajed T, Steele MA, Plastow GS, Wishart DS. Livestock metabolomics and the livestock metabolome: A systematic review. PLoS One 2017;12:1–26.

[84] Kenéz, Warnken T, Feige K, Huber K. Lower plasma trans-4-hydroxyproline and methionine sulfoxide levels are associated with insulin dysregulation in horses. BMC Vet Res 2018.

[85] Jacob SI, Murray KJ, Rendahl AK, Geor RJ, Schultz NE, McCue ME. Metabolic perturbations in Welsh Ponies with insulin dysregulation, obesity, and laminitis. J Vet Intern Med 2018:1–19.

[86] Carlos Eduardo Medina Torres. Equine Laminitis: a Tissue Microdialysis Study of Lamellar Bioenergetics. University of Queensland, 2014.

[87] Coleman MC, Whitfield-Cargile CM, Madrigal RG, Cohen ND. Comparison of the microbiome, metabolome, and lipidome of obese and non-obese horses. PLoS One 2019;14:1–17.

[88] Wyse CA, McNie KA, Tannahill VJ, Love S, Murray JK, Tannahil VJ, et al. Prevalence of obesity in riding horses in Scotland. Vet Rec 2008;162:590–1.

[89] Stephenson HM, Green MJ, Freeman SL. Prevalence of obesity in a population of horses in the UK. Vet Rec 2011;168:131–131.

[90] Equine Endocrinology Group. Recommendations for the Diagnosis and Treatment of Equine Metabolic Syndrome (EMS) 2016:https://sites.tufts.edu/equineendogroup/files/2016. https://sites.tufts.edu/equineendogroup/files/2016/11/2016-11-2-EMS-EEG-Final.pdf.

[91] Treiber KH, Kronfeld DS, Hess TM, Boston RC, Harris P a. Use of proxies and reference quintiles obtained from minimal model analysis for determination of insulin sensitivity and pancreatic beta-cell responsiveness in horses. Am J Vet Res 2005;66:2114–21.

[92] Pratt SE, Siciliano PD, Walston L. Variation of Insulin Sensitivity Estimates in Horses. J Equine Vet Sci 2009;29:507–12.

[93] Sherwin RS, Kramer KJ, Tobin JD, Insel PA, Liljenquist JE, Berman M, et al. A model of the kinetics of insulin in man. J Clin Invest 1974;53:1481–92.

[94] DeFronzo RA, Tobin JD, Andres R. Glucose clamp technique: a method for quantifying insulin secretion and resistance. Am J Physiol Metab 1979;237:E214.

[95] Pratt SE, Geor RJ, McCutcheon LJ. Repeatability of 2 methods for assessment of insulin sensitivity and glucose dynamics in horses. J Vet Intern Med 2005;19:883–8.

[96] Eiler H, Frank N, Andrews FM, Oliver JW, Fecteau KA. Physiologic assessment of blood glucose homeostasis via combined intravenous glucose and insulin testing in horses. Am J Vet Res 2005;66:1598–604.

[97] Bertin FR, Sojka-Kritchevsky JE. Comparison of a 2-step insulin-response test to conventional insulin-sensitivity testing in horses. Domest Anim Endocrinol 2013;44:19–25.

[98] Bamford NJ, Potter SJ, Baskerville CL, Harris PA, Bailey SR. Influence of dietary restriction and low-intensity exercise on weight loss and insulin sensitivity in obese equids. J Vet Intern Med 2019;33:280–6.

[99] Morgan RA, Keen JA, McGowan CM. Treatment of equine metabolic syndrome: A clinical case series. Equine Vet J 2016;48:422–6.

[100] Dugdale AHA, Curtis GC, Cripps P, Harris PA, Argo MM. Effect of dietary restriction on body condition, composition and welfare of overweight and obese pony mares. Equine Vet J 2010;42:600–10.

[101] Gill JC, Pratt-Phillips SE, Mansmann R, Siciliano PD. Weight Loss Management in Client-Owned Horses. J Equine Vet Sci 2016;39:80–9.

[102] Trussardi Fayh AP, Lopes AL, Fernandes PR, Reischak-Oliveira A, Friedman R. Impact of weight loss with or without exercise on abdominal fat and insulin resistance in obese individuals: a

randomised clinical trial. Br J Nutr 2013;110:486–92.

[103] Bird SR, Hawley JA. Update on the effects of physical activity on insulin sensitivity in humans. BMJ Open Sport Exerc Med 2017;2:1–26.

[104] Pedersen BK, Febbraio MA. Muscles, exercise and obesity: Skeletal muscle as a secretory organ. Nat Rev Endocrinol 2012;8:457–65.

[105] Brotto M, Johnson ML. Endocrine Crosstalk Between Muscle and Bone. Curr Osteoporos Rep 2014;12:135–41.

[106] Suagee JK, Corl BA, Wearn JG, Crisman M V., Hulver MW, Geor RJ, et al. Effects of the Insulin-Sensitizing Drug Pioglitazone and Lipopolysaccharide Administration on Insulin Sensitivity in Horses. J Vet Intern Med 2011;25:356–64.

[107] Tinworth KD, Edwards S, Harris PA, Sillence MN, Hackett LP, Noble GK. Pharmacokinetics of metformin after enteral administration in insulin-resistant ponies. Am J Vet Res 2010;71:1201–6.

[108] Durham AE. Metformin in equine metabolic syndrome: an enigma or a dead duck? Vet J 2012;191:17–8.

[109] Durham AE, Rendle DI, Newton JE. The effect of metformin on measurements of insulin sensitivity and beta cell response in 18 horses and ponies with insulin resistance. Equine Vet J 2008;40:493–500.

[110] Tinworth KD, Boston RC, Harris PA, Sillence MN, Raidal SL, Noble GK. The effect of oral metformin on insulin sensitivity in insulin-resistant ponies. Vet J 2012;191:79–84.

[111] Rendle DI, Rutledge F, Hughes KJ, Heller J, Durham AE. Effects of metformin hydrochloride on blood glucose and insulin responses to oral dextrose in horses. Equine Vet J 2013;45:751–4.

[112] Meier A, Reiche D, de Laat M, Pollitt C, Walsh D, Sillence M. The sodium-glucose co-transporter 2 inhibitor velagliflozin reduces hyperinsulinemia and prevents laminitis in insulin-dysregulated ponies. PLoS One 2018;13:1–13.

[113] Frank N, Sommardahl CS, Eiler H, Webb LL, Denhart JW, Boston RC. Effects of oral administration of levothyroxine sodium on concentrations of plasma lipids, concentration and composition of very-low-density lipoproteins, and glucose dynamics in healthy adult mares. Am J Vet Res 2005;66:1032–8.

[114] Ho JE, Larson MG, Vasan RS, Ghorbani A, Cheng S, Rhee EP, et al. Metabolite profiles during oral glucose challenge. Diabetes 2013;62:2689–98.

[115] Mangge H, Summers KL, Meinitzer A, Zelzer S, Almer G, Prassl R, et al. Obesity-related dysregulation of the Tryptophan-Kynurenine metabolism: Role of age and parameters of the metabolic syndrome. Obesity 2014;22:195–201.

[116] Lundquist I, Panagiotidis G, Stenstrom A. Effect of L-DOPA administration on islet monoamine oxidase activity and glucose-induced insulin release in the mouse. Pancreas 1991;6:522–7.

[117] Boyd AE, Lebovitz HE, Feldman JM. Endocrine function and glucose metabolism in patients with parkinson's disease and their alteration by L-dopa. J Clin Endocrinol Metab 1971;33:829–37.

[118] Millington WR, Dybdal NO, Dawson R, Manzini C, Mueller GP. Equine Cushing's Disease: Differential Regulation of β-Endorphin Processing in Tumors of the Intermediate Pituitary. Endocrinology 1988;123:1598–604.

[119] Lipman IJ, Boykin ME, Flora RE. Glucose intolerance in parkinson's disease. J Chronic Dis 1974.

[120] Santiago JA, Potashkin JA. Shared dysregulated pathways lead to Parkinson's disease and diabetes. Trends Mol Med 2013;19:176–86.

[121] Paapstel K, Kals J, Eha J, Tootsi K, Ottas A, Piir A, et al. Metabolomic profiles of lipid metabolism, arterial stiffness and hemodynamics in male coronary artery disease patients. IJC Metab Endocr 2016;11:13–8.

[122] Wooldridge AA, Waguespack RW, Schwartz DD, Venugopal CS, Eades SC, Beadle RE. Vasorelaxation responses to insulin in laminar vessel rings from healthy, lean horses. Vet J 2014;202:83–8.

[123] Moore JL, Siciliano PD, Pratt-Phillips SE. Effects of Diet Versus Exercise on Morphometric Measurements, Blood Hormone Concentrations, and Oral Sugar Test Response in Obese Horses. J Equine Vet Sci 2019;78:38–45.

[124] Gordon ME, McKeever KH, Betros CL, Manso Filho HC. Exercise-induced alterations in plasma concentrations of ghrelin, adiponectin, leptin, glucose, insulin, and cortisol in horses. Vet J 2007;173:532–40.

[125] de Laat MA, Hampson BA, Sillence MN, Pollitt CC. Sustained, Low-Intensity Exercise Achieved by a Dynamic Feeding System Decreases Body Fat in Ponies. J Vet Intern Med 2016;30:1732–8.

[126] Potter SJ, Bamford NJ, Harris PA, Bailey SR. Comparison of weight loss, with or without dietary restriction and exercise, in Standardbreds, Andalusians and mixed breed ponies. J Equine Vet Sci 2013;33:339.

[127] Quinn RW, Burk AO, Hartsock TG, Petersen ED, Whitley NC, Treiber KH, et al. Insulin Sensitivity in Thoroughbred Geldings: Effect of Weight Gain, Diet, and Exercise on Insulin Sensitivity in Thoroughbred Geldings. J Equine Vet Sci 2008;28:728–38.

[128] Carter R a, McCutcheon LJ, George L a, Smith TL, Frank N, Geor RJ. Effects of diet-induced weight gain on insulin sensitivity and plasma hormone and lipid concentrations in horses. Am J Vet Res 2009;70:1250–8.

[129] Floyd JC, Fajans SS, Conn JW, Knopf RF, Rull J. Stimulation of insulin secretion by amino acids. J Clin Invest 1966;45:1487–502.

[130] Bode-Böger SM. Effect of L-arginine supplementation on NO production in man. Eur J Clin Pharmacol 2006;62:91–9.

[131] Pieper GM. Review of alterations in endothelial nitric oxide production in diabetes: Protective role of arginine on endothelial dysfunction. Hypertension 1998;31:1047–60.

[132] Cave MC, Hurt RT, Frazier TH, Matheson PJ, Garrison RN, McClain CJ, et al. Obesity, inflammation, and the potential application of pharmaconutrition. Nutr Clin Pract 2008;23:16–34.

[133] Eid HMA, Reims H, Arnesen H, Kjeldsen SE, Lyberg T, Seljeflot I. Decreased levels of asymmetric dimethylarginine during acute hyperinsulinemia. Metabolism 2007;56:464–9.

[134] Wallace M, Morris C, O'Grada CM, Ryan M, Dillon ET, Coleman E, et al. Relationship between the lipidome, inflammatory markers and insulin resistance. Mol BioSyst 2014;10:1586–95.

[135] Gorres KL, Raines RT. Prolyl 4-hydroxylase. vol. 45. 2010.

[136] Castro GD, Castro JA. Hydroxyproline reaction with free radicals generated during benzoyl peroxide catalytic decomposition of carbon tetrachloride Structure of reaction products formed. Amino Acids 1996;10:283–94.

[137] Milić S, Bogdanović Pristov J, Mutavdžić D, Savić A, Spasić M, Spasojević I. The relationship of physicochemical properties to the antioxidative activity of free amino acids in fenton system. Environ Sci Technol 2015;49:4245–54.

[138] Xie B, Waters MJ, Schirra HJ. Investigating Potential Mechanisms of Obesity by Metabolomics. J Biomed Biotechnol 2012;2012:1–10.

[139] Seiler SE, Martin OJ, Noland RC, Slentz DH, DeBalsi KL, Ilkayeva OR, et al. Obesity and lipid stress inhibit carnitine acetyltransferase activity. J Lipid Res 2014;55:635–44.

[140] Talenezhad N, Mohammadi M, Ramezani-Jolfaie N, Mozaffari-Khosravi H, Salehi-Abargouei A. Effects of L-carnitine supplementation on weight loss and body composition: A systematic review and meta-analysis of 37 randomized controlled clinical trials with dose-response analysis. Clin Nutr ESPEN 2020;37:9–23.

[141] Xu Y, Jiang W, Chen G, Zhu W, Ding W, Ge Z, et al. L-carnitine treatment of insulin resistance: A systematic review and meta-analysis. Adv Clin Exp Med 2017;26:333–8.

[142] Schmengler U, Ungru J, Boston R, Coenen M, Vervuert I. Effects of l-carnitine supplementation on body weight losses and metabolic profile in obese and insulin-resistant ponies during a 14-week body weight reduction programme. Livest Sci 2013;155:301–7.

[143] Van Weyenberg S, Buyse J, Janssens GPJ. Increased plasma leptin through l-carnitine supplementation is associated with an enhanced glucose tolerance in healthy ponies. J Anim Physiol Anim Nutr 2009;93:203–8.

[144] Floegel A, Stefan N, Yu Z, Mühlenbruch K, Drogan D, Joost HG, et al. Identification of serum metabolites associated with risk of type 2 diabetes using a targeted metabolomic approach. Diabetes 2013;62:639–48.

[145] Rhee EP, Cheng S, Larson MG, Walford GA, Lewis GD, McCabe E, et al. Lipid profiling identifies a triacylglycerol signature of insulin resistance and improves diabetes prediction in humans. J Clin Invest 2011;121:1402–11.

[146] Ding M, Rexrode KM. A review of lipidomics of cardiovascular disease highlights the importance of isolating lipoproteins. Metabolites 2020;10:1–13.

[147] Felig P. The glucose-alanine cycle. Metabolism 1973;22:179–207.

[148] Consoli A, Nurjhan N, Reilly JJ, Bier DM, Gerich JE. Mechanism of increased gluconeogenesis in noninsulin-dependent diabetes mellitus. Role of alterations in systemic, hepatic, and muscle lactate and alanine metabilism. J Clin Invest 1990;86:2038–45.

Acknowledgements

I am thankful to **Professor Karsten Feige** for the opportunity to conduct this project, but I especially acknowledge how, alongside **Professor Korinna Huber** and **Professor Klaus Jung**, he provided a constructive and encouraging atmosphere, granting me much freedom and support. I appreciate that scientific integrity and respect for the animals we study were the pillars of my scientific education. I am very grateful to my supervisors for inspiring me in my work and beyond.

I would like to thank **Professor Martin Sillence**, **Alexandra Meier, PhD**, and **Dr. Dania Reiche** for the fruitful and pleasant collaboration as well as for the enriching feedback.

Special thanks to **Dr. Tobias Warnken, PhD**, without whom this project would never have come about, for his constant help and always sympathetic ear.

The completion of this work would not have been possible without the everlasting support of **Lisa Weber**, **Julia Gersch**, **Florian Frers** and **Anne Grob**. Thank you for listening to my complaints, believing in me, and accompanying me on this journey.

Thank you to **Dr. Björn Steinbjörnsson** and **Professor Wolfgang Leibold** for their dedicated care for the horses and help during the experiments.

Many thanks to the **HGNI**, especially to **Tanja Czeslik** and **Dr. Tina Selle**, and to all those who were involved in the organization of events and lectures. I greatly appreciated the PhD program and the effort put into it.

Thanks also to **all my colleagues and friends** for their help and moral support, for the laughs and the wine.

Finally, I would like to express my gratitude to my **family** for their support and understanding. I know that they are always there for me.

www.ingramcontent.com/pod-product-compliance
Ingram Content Group UK Ltd.
Pitfield, Milton Keynes, MK11 3LW, UK
UKHW021959190726
13853UKWH00004B/1627

9 783736 974265